INTRODUCTION TO
Health professions

INTRODUCTION TO
Health professions

Edited by

ANNE S. ALLEN, M.A., O.T.R.

Assistant Professor, Occupational Therapy Division,
School of Allied Medical Professions,
The Ohio State University,
Columbus, Ohio

First edition edited by

RUTH F. ODGERS, B.A.
BURNESS G. WENBERG, M.S., R.D.

Second edition

Illustrated

The C. V. Mosby Company

Saint Louis   1976

Second edition

Copyright © 1976 by The C. V. Mosby Company

All rights reserved. No part of this book may be reproduced in any manner without written permission of the publisher.

Previous edition copyrighted 1972

Printed in the United States of America

Distributed in Great Britain by Henry Kimpton, London

Library of Congress Cataloging in Publication Data

Main entry under title:

Introduction to health professions.

    Bibliography: p.
    Includes index.
    1. Medicine—Vocational guidance.   I. Allen, Anne S., 1923-   II. Title. [DNLM: 1. Health occupations. W21 I61]
R690.I57   1976   610.69   75-31827
ISBN 0-8016-0112-6

GW/M/M 9 8 7 6 5 4 3 2 1

Contributors

Anne S. Allen, M.A., O.T.R.
Assistant Professor, Occupational Therapy Division,
School of Allied Medical Professions,
The Ohio State University

Philip W. Ballinger, M.S., R.T.(ARRT)
Director, Radiologic Technology Division,
School of Allied Medical Professions,
The Ohio State University

Mary Alice Beetham, M.S.P.H.
Assistant Professor, Health Education, and Coordinator,
Advisory Committee, Health Education Extension Services,
The Ohio State University

John W. Black, Ph.D.
Regents Professor, Speech and Hearing Science,
Department of Communication,
The Ohio State University

Monica V. Brown, B.A.
Director, Health Careers of Ohio—Operation MEDIHC,
College of Medicine, The Ohio State University

Marjorie L. Brunner, M.S., M.T.(ASCP)
Assistant Professor, Medical Technology Division,
School of Allied Medical Professions,
The Ohio State University

J. Robert Bullock, R.T.(ARRT)
Director, Radiologic Technology Program,
Mt. Carmel Medical Center, Columbus, Ohio

Contributors

John E. Burke, Ph.D.

Director, Medical Communications Division,
School of Allied Medical Professions,
The Ohio State University

Clarence R. Cole, Ph.D., D.V.M.

Regents Professor and former Dean,
College of Veterinary Medicine,
The Ohio State University

Mae M. Davis, M.S.W., ACSW

Assistant Director, Medical Social Service Department,
The Ohio State University Hospitals

James P. Dearing, B.S.

Extracorporeal Circulation Technology Program,
Medical University of South Carolina,
Charleston, South Carolina

William C. Dew, D.D.S.

Associate Dean, Secretary, and Professor, College of Dentistry,
The Ohio State University

George L. Fite, M.D.

Bethesda, Maryland; formerly Division of Scientific Publications,
American Medical Association, Chicago, Illinois

O. Theodore Haaland, B.A.(ARRT)

Universal Hospital Services, Inc.,
Minneapolis, Minnesota

Katherine L. Kisker, R.N., M.S.

Instructor, School of Nursing,
The Ohio State University

David A. Knapp, Ph.D.

Professor, Pharmacy Administration, School of Pharmacy,
University of Maryland, Baltimore, Maryland

James R. Kreutzfeld, B.F.A.

Director, Medical Illustration Division,
School of Allied Medical Professions,
The Ohio State University

Thelma Lang, R.N., C.R.N.A.

Director, Nurse Anesthesiology Division,
School of Allied Medical Professions,
The Ohio State University

Elizabeth J. Laschinger, M.S.W., ACSW

Assistant Professor, Department of Social Work,
Capital University, Columbus, Ohio

Barbara McCool, M.H.A., Ph.D.

Associate Professor, Department of Health Administration,
Duke University, Durham, North Carolina

William F. Munsey, D.P.M.

Clinical Instructor, College of Medicine,
The Ohio State University

James F. Noe, M.A.

Assistant to the Dean and College Secretary, College of Optometry,
The Ohio State University

Melanie Moersch Pariser, M.S., R.R.A.

Assistant Director, Medical Records Administration Division,
School of Allied Medical Professions,
The Ohio State University

Frank M. Pierson, M.A., L.P.T.

Director, Physical Therapy Division,
School of Allied Medical Professions,
The Ohio State University

Mitzi Prosser, B.F.A.

Instructor, Medical Illustration Division,
School of Allied Medical Professions,
The Ohio State University

Nancy M. Reynolds, D.D.S.

Professor and Director, Division of Dental Hygiene,
College of Dentistry,
The Ohio State University

Ethelrine Shaw, R.N., M.S.N.
Associate Professor, Maternity Nursing,
School of Nursing,
The Ohio State University

James A. Visconti, Ph.D.
Associate Professor, College of Pharmacy,
The Ohio State University;
Director, Drug Information Center,
The Ohio State University Hospitals

Burness G. Wenberg, M.S., R.D.
Associate Professor and Coordinator, Undergraduate Dietetic Curriculum,
Department of Food Science and Human Nutrition,
College of Human Ecology, Michigan State University,
East Lansing, Michigan

J. Scott Worley, M.A., O.T.R.
Assistant Professor, Department of Occupational Therapy,
School of Allied Health and Social Professions,
East Carolina University,
Greenville, North Carolina

Preface

In the course of teaching many hundreds of undergraduate college students about the various health professions, many questions and areas of confusion repeatedly arose. To students who have not come from families with personal or professional ties to the health field, the whole area holds a mystery both unwarranted and self-defeating. It was with the purpose of dispelling some of this mystery and showing the variety of professional pursuits these fields offer, how to prepare for them, and what to expect of them that Burness Wenberg developed the course "Introduction to Health Professions" at The Ohio State University. This course formed the basis for the first edition of this book.

In their preface to the first edition, Odgers and Wenberg wrote:

> This book is designed to provide educational and occupational information for a wide variety of health careers at a time when more and more young people are urgently needed in almost every area of health service. It is intended to show how the health professional functions in his job, what is necessary by way of education and training, and what opportunities for employment are available. It is hoped that it may prove equally useful as a textbook or as a resource for vocational counseling.

It has been my privilege to teach the course to hundreds of students, who have assisted in this revision through their questions, comments, and suggestions. All chapters have been written by practitioners, educators, or planners in health fields. All contributors are closely associated with the problems of attracting competent, motivated persons to the health professions, teaching them, and assisting their plans for effective service. Most authors had trouble dealing with the universal question of salaries and compensation. Some chose to ignore the question, others cited ranges. It should be pointed out that most baccalaureate health practitioners start at similar salaries within a given *geographic location*. There are great variations between locations such as the Midwest and the West Coast and between urban and rural settings.

The decision concerning the professions to include in a book of this size were made on the basis of two criteria: (1) that the profession's educational program be established in significant numbers of schools at the baccalaureate level or above and (2) that it be involved with either direct services to patients or health information systems. Because of its parallel with and impact on human health care, we chose to include veterinary medicine. We regretfully chose not to continue the chapter on environmental sanitation in this second edition because of the constraints of space and the second criterion.

The appendixes are designed to give quick information in reference form concerning the length of time necessary to complete training programs, the titles of related health vocations, some manpower statistics, and professional organizations.

Chapter 1 deals with the meaning of "profession" and the responsibilities that accompany that designation and affect the lives of practitioners everywhere. Within each field there is a tendency to subdivide as the knowledge and skills expand. This process gives the responsibility for less demanding operations to people with less training and creates ladders within the field that are useful and attractive for persons wishing to serve in a helping capacity but not wishing to commit themselves to the educational programs and practices of professional service. It is hoped that Appendix B will prove helpful to students seeking these alternative goals.

Grateful acknowledgment is made to Kay Buckey White and Barbara Martin for their thoughtful contributions to the first edition. Some of their material has been retained and revised in this edition.

Further acknowledgment is due to Marjorie Brunner, who was largely responsible for the revision of the appendixes, and to Robert J. Atwell, Carolyn Burnett, and J. Hutchinson Williams for their helpful comments and manuscript suggestions. To all the contributing authors and the previous editors, Ruth Odgers and Burness Wenberg, my thanks.

Anne S. Allen

Contents

1 **Development of the health professions,** 1
   Anne S. Allen

2 **Dental hygiene,** 9
   Nancy M. Reynolds

3 **Dentistry,** 14
   William C. Dew

4 **Dietetics,** 21
   Burness G. Wenberg

5 **Extracorporeal circulation technology,** 31
   James P. Dearing

6 **Health education,** 36
   Mary Alice Beetham

7 **Hospital and health services administration,** 41
   Barbara McCool

8 **Medical communications,** 47
   John E. Burke

9 **Medical illustration,** 55
   Mitzi Prosser and James R. Kreutzfeld

10 **Medical record administration,** 60
   Melanie Moersch Pariser

11 **Medical technology,** 71
   Marjorie L. Brunner

12 **Medicine,** 81
   George L. Fite

13 **Nursing and related programs,** 91
   Nursing, 91
   Katherine L. Kisker

Nurse anesthesiology, 98
Thelma Lang

Nurse-midwifery, 101
Ethelrine Shaw

14 Occupational therapy, 104
J. Scott Worley

15 Optometry, 112
James F. Noe

16 Pharmacy, 118
David A. Knapp and James A. Visconti

17 Physical therapy, 124
Frank M. Pierson

18 Physician's assistant, 133
Monica V. Brown

19 Podiatry, 137
William F. Munsey

20 Radiologic technology, 141
J. Robert Bullock and Philip W. Ballinger

21 Respiratory therapy, 148
O. Theodore Haaland

22 Social work, 156

Medical social work, 156
Mae M. Davis

Social work in mental health settings, 161
Elizabeth J. Laschinger

23 Speech and hearing science, 165
John W. Black

24 Veterinary medicine, 173
Clarence R. Cole

Appendixes

    A Calendar of health careers, 184

    B Related health occupations, 187

    C Supply of active formally trained selected health personnel, 189

    D Professional organizations where further information may be obtained, 190

INTRODUCTION TO
Health professions

Chapter 1
Development of the health professions
Anne S. Allen

The health professions as they exist today have developed in response to the demands of the technological and population expansions of the first part of the twentieth century. This rapid and enthusiastic growth within the health care family has produced problems that recapitulate those of human families in terms of adolescent turmoil and sibling rivalry. This has been demonstrated by the growing pains of professional organizations and by interdisciplinary quarrels over areas of patient care. That the new professions are showing signs of maturing into responsible components of the health care system is attributable to three factors: the impact of professionalism, the demand of the public for quality care, and the growing legislative support for health care.

IMPACT OF PROFESSIONALISM

Most groups of health practitioners either have already or are proceeding to professionalize their services. The professionalization of an occupation affects career choice through the selection of students. It also affects their education and the focus of their future energies. Professionalization should therefore be examined in terms of its historical development and its benefits and responsibilities.

The practice of medicine has always been identified as a profession and was one of the original three professions established during the rise of the universities in the Middle Ages, the other two being law and theology. There are some today who believe that these three are still the only professions and that others merely aspire to a status that is fundamentally beyond them. In his writings during the early part of this century, Abraham Flexner developed the following criteria for professions. He wrote that professions must be intellectual in their judgmental components, possessing a large body of knowledge unique to their own pursuits; they must be practical in that this knowledge can be applied to real situations; they must possess teachable techniques that can be used for problem solving; they must be organized into associations committed to the regulation, education, and protection of their members; and they must be governed by altruism.

It is probably because of the struggle on the part of so many skilled, helpful, and well-motivated people to professionalize their endeavors that McGlothlin has added a further criterion: a profession must "deal with matters of urgency and significance." Only the purest of academicians today would limit the professions to the original three.

If a group of practitioners establish their credentials according to these criteria and if they are engaged in promoting the state of well-being known as health, they are recognized as health professionals. The concept is broadened significantly by our current disinclination to define health merely as the absence of disease. There is universal acceptance of the World Health Organization's broader concept of health, which defines it as a state of functional well-being having the physical, psychological, and social aspects of the individual in equilibrium.

In any discussion of health professions their debt to the traditional professional model of medicine must be acknowledged. Just as the business and administrative professions owe much to the original profession of law and the teaching professions owe much to theology, so the health professions relate to medicine. From this field they have learned their research techniques, their model of professional organization, and their responsiveness to human need.

It is the adherence to Flexner's criteria for professions that gives rise to many of the problems of the new as well as the more established health professions. Because of their unique bodies of knowledge, these professions must constantly evaluate their bases for practice and revise them through research. Practitioners must teach this information to students and experienced practitioners alike and must further disseminate new knowledge through journals and other publications. The professional organizations that "regulate, educate, and protect" their members require significant amounts of energy and money from their members in order to do their job. They must also at times answer charges of guildism and restraint of trade. Because of their concern with urgent matters of human need, they have worked to design certifying procedures that will protect the public from opportunistic charlatans. In their service to the public they must accept governmental assistance while avoiding governmental control.

Certifying procedures have two components. One component is concerned with establishing, usually by examination, the credentials both of the individual and of his educational institution. The other component deals with what the individual is taught.

Establishing credentials

Professionals who serve the public must demonstrate qualifications to perform that service in such a way that people needing to buy the service can do so with the assurance that they will receive what they are paying for. The professional's ability to serve is evidenced by (1) the quality of the professional school attended and (2) personal knowledge and abilities. The school's qualifications to teach the professional program (whether medicine, occupational therapy, dental hygiene, or another area of health care) are determined through the process of *ac-*

creditation. As part of the accreditation process, a school's curriculum, faculty, and facilities are examined by a committee representing educators and members of the particular profession according to a process set forth by the professional association. Attending an accredited school ensures students of the integrity of their preparation. Attending a non-accredited school makes future employability doubtful. The professional's own personal knowledge and abilities are further attested to by *certification, licensure,* or *registration* within the profession.

In some professions a certificate from an accredited school makes the graduate eligible for membership in that profession without further examination. Members of other professions are additionally either licensed or registered. *Licensure* is a state-controlled process in which professionals sit for an examination that determines their eligibility for a state license to practice. Reciprocity exists among many but not all states.

Although occasionally it is simply a procedure, the process of *registration* is usually controlled by individual professional organizations, which sometimes require examination and usually require graduation from an accredited school. (Some professions, in the interest both of freer entry into the profession and of career mobility, are allowing persons with equivalent experience to take the qualifying examinations. At this time, it is difficult to establish equivalency.)

A student who wants to enter a professional field must investigate and follow the certification procedures of that field. The procedures have been designed to safeguard the public by ensuring that doctors, nurses, therapists, and other health care practitioners are qualified to practice. Further safeguards are being introduced in the form of continuing education requirements for continued certification.

Education of health professionals

Important trends in the education of health professionals have included the shift from hospital-based programs to those established in universities and from apprenticeships to balanced curriculums. This shift took place in part because of the need to have the costs of education paid for by those receiving it. As training programs moved into educational institutions, the responsibility for determining the number and quality of individuals entering the profession fell to the professional schools. As a result, professional schools became actively engaged in student recruitment and admission, and this in turn involved establishing criteria for selection. As the selection process evolved, the competition for places in entering classes increased. The inevitable result was that the pressure to make career choices extended downward to ever earlier ages, so that qualifications could be built and the selection criteria met.

The process of professional education in a liberal arts setting has its own confusions. Trade and vocational schools, like many of the early hospital programs that trained nurses and technicians, are quite frankly technical in nature and can provide "understanding of fundamental principles of technologies and the development of skills and techniques." A university, however, is an institution dedicated to the purpose of training minds. Attainment of technical and mechanical skills is secondary to the acquisition of knowledge and mental discipline.* A professional school must combine the two philosophies, assisting students to acquire knowledge and discipline while at the same time educating them to understand technological principles and to develop skills and techniques for applying theory to practice.

Students who wish to enter a health profession, then, must be able to pursue knowledge and discipline their minds according to the philosophy of liberal arts education, while at the same time acquiring the necessary professional skills and techniques. Needless to say, the two aspects are seldom perfectly balanced in individuals, and fortunately so. It is the difference in these abilities that produces the different kinds of professionals—researchers, healers, teachers, clinicians, planners, etc.

In contrast to the varying interests and abilities of its students, each profession must maintain basically similar programs that include the essentials of education balanced in such a way that students can acquire the prerequisites during their preprofessional education and pursue their professional studies through a carefully planned mixture of academic and clinical experience. The development of the *essentials*, or standard educational requirements, is the responsibility of the professional organization. The essentials are usually developed by a committee of the association, approved by the entire association, and supervised by a different committee.

DEMAND OF THE PUBLIC FOR QUALITY CARE

In an address at the convocation of entering medical students at the Ohio State University in 1974, Dr. John Cooper, president of the Association of American Medical Colleges, said, "The increased demand for care comes from the very success of modern scientific medicine in preventing, diagnosing, and curing disease. The public has learned through mass media what is now possible and they want the advances we have achieved...."

The health professions have been responding to the demand for more and better services by increasing student enrollments in order to produce more practitioners. Two further and perhaps more significant responses have been the encouragement of continuing education and the development of the team concept.

---

*Discipline may be defined as a branch of knowledge or learning and also as training that develops self-control, character, or orderliness and efficiency.

Continuing education

Technological advances through research and the development of new techniques and equipment have made many once-trusted medical procedures obsolete. New procedures have been developed. For example, entire wings of hospitals, together with their highly specialized personnel, were restructured and diverted to other needs as the Salk/Sabin polio vaccines virtually eliminated poliomyelitis and the number of such patients was reduced almost to zero. New advances in heart surgery have necessitated the further education of many surgeons and operating room personnel. In addition, people wishing to reenter a health care field after a period of inactivity (for example, women who have been at home for several years with young children) create a demand for short courses and programs that will help them to reacquire lost skills and keep abreast of advancing knowledge.

Opportunities for continuing education are available through universities and other institutions, through conferences and workshops sponsored by professional organizations, sometimes through correspondence courses, and always through professional journals. It is the responsibility of all health professionals to maintain and enhance their own levels of competence.

Team concept

It is obvious that the ultimate in health care cannot be delivered by one person. In the first place, it would be impossible for one person to know all there is to know about medicine and its related technologies. Second, even if one individual could know it all, there would be neither the time nor the energy to apply this knowledge. Consequently, the concept of the health team has been developed, and it has met with varying degrees of acceptance by health practitioners. In the report of the conference on the interrelationships of educational programs for health professionals, held in October of 1972 at the National Academy of Sciences in Washington, D.C., Pellegrino wrote, "There is no such thing as 'the team' in health care. Instead, there are a *large number* of health teams, dedicated to varying purposes. . . . The purpose of a team approach is to optimize the special contribution in skills and knowledge of the team members so that the needs of the persons served can be met more efficiently, competently, and more considerately than would be possible by independent and individual action."

Pellegrino defines two types of teams, functional and patient centered. Both are transitory and both depend on the problem to be solved, whether individual, family, or community. Functional teams are those whose personnel depend on the nature of the problem (for example, the coronary care team, the nursing team, the mental health team, etc.). Patient-centered teams are made up in terms of closeness of patient contact. Pellegrino further divides the patient-centered teams into three categories.

6 Introduction to health professions

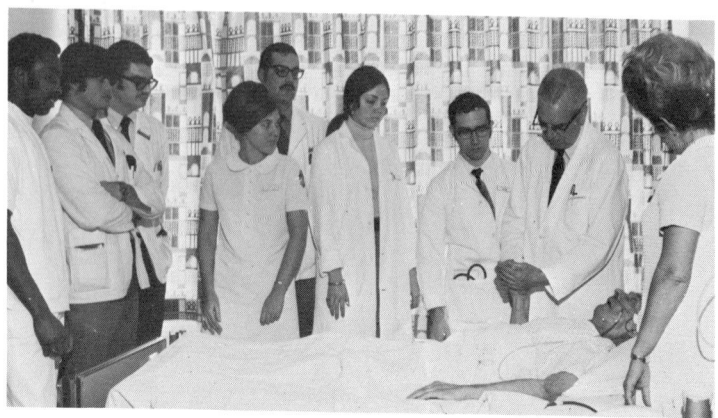

Fig. 1. The combined skills of many professionals contribute to modern health care.

1. The patient care team is made up of people "who jointly provide needed services that bring them into direct personal and physical contact with the patient and which are part of his personal and individualized program of management.... These are the people who lay hands directly on the patient, have the most sustained contact with him as a person, rather than with a part of him, and must experience with him the joy of cure and the burden of failure and death." Doctors, nurses, therapists, etc. comprise these teams.

2. The medical care team is made up of people who provide "essential back-up services for the patient care teams ... not in close continual contact with the patient ... some deal transiently on a personal basis with the patient ... for a short interval. Others do not work with the patient personally. They deal with a part of the patient—his sputum, urine, x-rays, medication and so forth." These team members are, for example, pathologists, radiologic technologists, medical technologists, and pharmacists.

3. The health care team is made up of persons who are the "most distantly related to the individual patients and usually have as their concern the entire community. Such teams concentrate on the health of the aggregate, the delivery of all services, their availability ... the costs of care, the distribution of resources ... the regulation of quality ... the production of manpower ... (this group includes) public health officers, hospital administrators, health educators, bio-medical engineers, sanitarians, etc."

If we accept the team concept, we must recognize its changing nature. Teams continually dissolve, and members regroup in order to meet special problems. Teams are discussed here not only because of their effect on the quality of health care but also because of the influence that many educators feel they have on the educational process and on a student's choice of a field of health care. (See Fig. 1.)

LEGISLATIVE SUPPORT FOR HEALTH CARE

Early legislation in the field of health care provided only for such urgent needs as those of dependent children, the blind, and the severely handicapped. More recently, Congress and the state legislatures have enacted laws that appropriate funds for three general purposes: to pay for services, to educate practitioners and consumers of health care, and to encourage research.

At present, members of most health professions are involved in various ways with legislated components of health care. Within the last fifteen years several laws have been passed by the federal government to accomplish specific purposes.
1. Medicare and Medicaid have been added to the Social Security Act to extend health care benefits to those over 65 years of age and to those under 65 who are medically indigent. The Professional Standards Review Organization was added more recently (1972) and provides a structure for review of the quality of services delivered.
2. The Health Manpower Acts have provided funds for building educational facilities, supporting basic professional education, and funding special projects and traineeships.
3. The Regional Medical Programs have made available money to combat the illnesses related to heart disease, cancer, and stroke.
4. Comprehensive Health Planning has supported health care planning within the community.
5. The National Institutes of Health supports research projects.
6. The Hill-Burton Act made money available for hospital construction.
7. The Health Maintenance Organization Act (1973) provided a five-year program of federal subsidies to prepaid group practices.

In addition, there has been federal and state legislative activity in the areas of abortion, contraception, use of human material for research, nursing home standards, occupational safety and health, organ transplatation, environmental hazards, and health insurance. There are presently at least six major proposals for national health insurance before the United States Congress, and there is a high probability that one of them will become law within the foreseeable future.

The quality and number of individuals involved in the health professions have grown significantly as a result of this governmental support. The growing public interest in health care for everyone will undoubtedly increase the demand for quality health care practitioners and at the same time encourage legislation providing payment for services.

SUMMARY

Today's health professions owe much to the traditions of medicine and nursing. The independence of the newer professions has been the logical outcome of their assumption of responsibility for specific areas of patient care, their technological advances, and their organizational responsibility for credentials, standards of practice, and public accountability. The demand for quality health care has fostered continuing education and interdisciplinary cooperation, the team approach. Throughout this development, legislation has played both enabling and regulatory roles.

REFERENCES

Columbus Tech bulletin 1973-1974, Columbus, Ohio, 1973, Columbus Technical Institute.

McGlothlin, W. J.: The professional schools, New York, 1974, Center for Applied Research in Education.

Pellegrino, E. D.: Interdisciplinary education in the health professions. In Educating for the health team, Washington, D.C., 1972, National Academy of Sciences–National Institute of Medicine.

SUGGESTED READINGS

Educating for the health team, Washington, D.C., 1972, National Academy of Sciences–National Institute of Medicine.

Hamburg, J., editor: Review of allied health education. I, Lexington, 1974, The University Press of Kentucky.

Weiss, L. B., and Spence, A. B.: A guide to the health professions, Cambridge, Mass., 1973, Office of Career Services and Off-Campus Learning, Harvard University.

Chapter 2

Dental hygiene

Nancy M. Reynolds

Dental hygiene is an auxiliary profession of dentistry and is one of the allied health professions. Its function, as defined by the American Dental Association (ADA), is to assist the members of the dental profession in providing oral health care to the public.

Dental hygiene is practiced by dental hygienists, who are sometimes called oral hygienists. They are licensed, professional oral health educators and clinical operators who, as auxiliaries to the dentist, use scientific methods in the control and prevention of oral disease, helping individuals and groups to develop and maintain optimum oral health. A dental hygienist's functions involve preventive dentistry, which includes dental health education (teaching methods of prevention to individual patients or to groups of individuals), and those clinical procedures (including oral prophylaxis) that are delegated by the dental profession.

BACKGROUND

Dental hygiene is a new profession when compared to dentistry, medicine, and nursing. Dr. Alfred C. Fones, a dentist, opened the first school for dental hygienists in 1913 in Bridgeport, Connecticut. He was convinced that general health could be improved by good oral health, and his main purpose in educating dental hygienists was to prepare them to work in the public schools in Bridgeport. In the schools, dental hygienists are oral health educators, teaching children proper oral hygiene habits to help them reduce dental decay and improve their oral health.

EDUCATIONAL PROGRAMS

Between 1957 and 1974 the number of accredited dental hygiene programs in the United States increased from thirty-four to one hundred and sixty, and many more programs are currently being developed. All dental hygiene programs must meet the standards established by the Council on Dental Education of the American Dental Association, which is composed of representatives from the American Dental Association, the American Association of Dental Examiners, and the American Association of Dental Schools. Admission requirements include the completion of a minimum of two academic years of college-level study at an accredited university, college, or junior college. Basic biology is usually a requirement for admission. Chemistry and mathematics are not always required, but it is usually recommended that students study these subjects either in high school or college. High school mathematics or test performance at a level indicating a basic knowledge of mathematics is often required.

Most schools also require that prospective dental hygiene students take the aptitude test administered by the American Dental Hygienists' Association. The test results are considered in conjunction with the applicant's other qualifications.

Traditionally, dental hygiene curricula were associated with schools of dentistry, but in recent years dental hygiene programs have been offered in two-year schools as well as in four-year colleges and universities. Various options are available to the prospective dental hygienist. Two-year junior or community colleges award an associate degree to those who successfully complete the program. Four-year colleges and universities may either offer certificates designating as graduate dental hygienists those who successfully complete the two-year program, or they may award baccalaureate degrees to those who complete the degree requirements plus the requirements for the dental hygiene program. The baccalaureate programs may integrate the university's arts and sciences requirements with an increasing emphasis on dental hygiene courses in each of the succeeding years, or the dental hygiene program may be concentrated in two of the four years of enrollment. A few programs in the United States are offered jointly with a college of education. In this type of program, students are required to do practice teaching in both general and dental health in elementary or secondary schools. On successful completion of this program, the graduate receives a bachelor of science degree in education and a teaching certificate from the state department of education. The combined education–dental hygiene program offers preparation for the dental hygiene profession as well as teacher preparation for dental health programs in schools, in the general community, and in schools of dental hygiene.

Some universities offer programs for the graduate dental hygienist leading to a master's degree. These may encompass dental hygiene, health education, public health, education, or the sciences. Among the institutions currently offering such programs are The Ohio State University, Columbus; Southern Illinois University, Carbondale; Columbia University, New York City; the University of Kentucky, Lexington; the University of Michigan, Ann Arbor; the University of Iowa, Iowa City; the University of Missouri–Kansas City School of Dentistry; and the University of Washington, Seattle.

CURRICULUM

Basic science requirements in dental hygiene programs include anatomy, microbiology, and physiology. Specific courses in English,

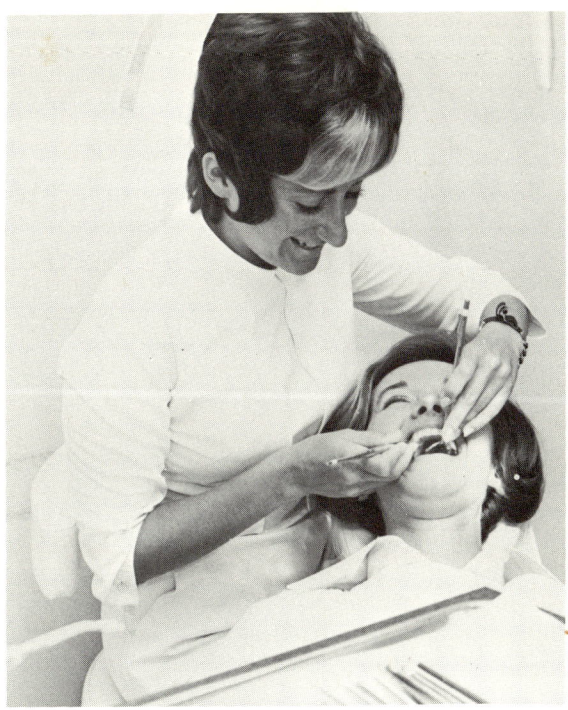

Fig. 2. Clinical application of dental hygiene procedures is an important part of the curriculum. A student performs an oral prophylaxis on a patient.

health education, nutrition, psychology, sociology, and speech are also required.

A dental hygiene curriculum also includes course work in anesthesia, chemistry, dental anatomy, dental materials, techniques of patient care and management, general pathology, oral histology and pathology, oral hygiene and oral hygiene programs for schools, pharmacology, practice management, public health, and radiography. In addition, most schools now include courses that teach functions formerly performed by dentists and only recently delegated to hygienists. Clinical experience is an important part of the dental hygiene curriculum, and courses in which students apply their skills and knowledge provide this experience. (See Fig. 2.)

LICENSING

In order to be licensed to practice, most dental hygienists take the written examination administered by the National Dental Hygiene Board, which is recognized in forty-seven states, the District of Columbia, Puerto Rico, and the Virgin Islands. Those states not using National

Board results are Arizona, Delaware, and New Jersey. In addition, most states require that the dental hygienist pass a practical examination.

FUNCTIONS OF THE DENTAL HYGIENIST AND CAREER OPPORTUNITIES

The dental hygienist is licensed to treat the patient in a private office or clinic by performing oral prophylaxis as well as other services for the patient. Dental hygienists may apply topical fluorides that make the surface of the tooth harder and less vulnerable to disease and may expose and develop radiographs of oral structures. The hygienist also assists the dentist by recognizing and reporting abnormalities of the oral cavity. A most important part of the dental hygienist's work involves educating patients regarding their own individual oral health needs and responsibilities in effectively preventing oral disease.

In many states, laws have been or are now being changed to permit expansion of the duties of this important dental auxiliary. Additional functions may include polishing restorations (fillings), placing sedative restorations, and taking impressions for making models of the teeth. Effective dental hygienists free dentists to perform only those services that require their skill and competence.

Dental hygienists who are employed in schools work directly to meet the foremost goal of the profession—education of the public. They are largely responsible for planning and executing that portion of the curriculum that pertains to their special field and for actually performing dental hygiene services if such treatment is provided in the school.

There are opportunities for employment in government institutions and programs, in industrial health programs, in research, in hospitals, and in the United States Army Medical Corps, where dental hygienists serve as commissioned officers. There are some positions available in foreign countries through the Peace Corps, with Project Hope, and with privately sponsored health care projects.

Although most dental hygienists are women, men are also welcome in the profession. Many male dental hygienists serve as health professionals in the armed services. Salaries paid to full-time dental hygienists vary considerably and depend on geographical location and the size and nature of the employing institution or facility as well as on the dental hygienist's training, experience, and professional responsibilities. In general, dental hygienists earn a beginning annual salary of $8,000 to $10,000.

PERSONAL QUALIFICATIONS

Those who are interested in the profession of dental hygiene should exhibit traits of personality and character that are consistent with the responsibilities they will assume on entering a health profession—responsibilities to the profession and to the public. Those who are unable or unwilling to give these responsibilities first priority in a professional situation should not enter the field of dental hygiene. Successful dental hygienists are sympathetic to people and their needs, are meticulous about detail, and are perfectionists in every facet of practice but patient in those instances where perfection cannot be achieved. They regard the profession of dentistry with respect.

PROFESSIONAL ORGANIZATIONS

The professional organization for dental hygienists is the American Dental Hygienists' Association. Affiliated with this organization is a students' counterpart, the Junior American Dental Hygienists' Association. Students are encouraged to join and participate in this organization so that they may learn about the professional organization that governs and protects them. Student members as well as professionals receive the *Journal of the American Dental Hygienists' Association*, the official publication of the organization.

SIGMA PHI ALPHA

Sigma Phi Alpha is the national dental hygiene honor society. Senior dental hygiene students who are outstanding in scholarship, leadership, and professional attitude are candidates for election to the society. The number of students elected annually from each class may not exceed 10% of the total number of students in the graduating class.

SUGGESTED READINGS

Motley, W. E.: Ethics, juris prudence
and history for the dental hygienist,
Philadelphia, 1972, Lea & Febiger.
Wilkins, E. M.: Clinical practice of
dental hygienist, ed. 3, Philadelphia,
1964, Lea & Febiger.

PROFESSIONAL ORGANIZATION WHERE FURTHER INFORMATION CAN BE OBTAINED

**American Dental Hygienists'
 Association**
211 East Chicago Avenue
Chicago, Illinois 60611

Chapter 3

Dentistry

William C. Dew

Dentistry is the profession that is concerned with maintaining the teeth and oral tissues in good health, preventing and treating dental diseases, and safeguarding the general health of the individual by detecting systemic disease in the oral tissues. It is a challenging profession that requires work with both the intellect and the hands. Dentistry affords the practitioner an opportunity to be artistic and skillful and offers independence, responsibility, authority, and opportunities for public service in a variety of situations.

HISTORY OF THE PROFESSION

The profession of dentistry shares a common origin with medicine. Many of the ancient medical documents and records contain references to dental diseases and their treatment. Egyptian records dating as far back as 3000 B.C. include sections on the treatment of dental diseases, although there is no mention of the removal of teeth or their replacement. The Phoenicians (1600-687 B.C.) were the first to devise and record methods of replacing missing teeth and retaining the replacements through the use of soldered gold bands or rivets. Improvements in this art were made by the Etruscans (753-300 B.C.), who lived in central Italy, and by the Greeks (377-162 B.C.), the Romans (450-218 B.C.), and the Arabians (700-1200 A.D.).

The first records of the separation of dentistry from the profession of medicine date from the thirteenth to the fifteenth centuries. Guy de Chauliac, a great surgeon of the Middle Ages, observed that operations on the teeth were properly the concern only of barbers and "dentatores." He made it clear that the "dentatores" of the fourteenth century were more than mere tooth pullers, for they treated diseases of the teeth and surrounding tissues as well as the scant knowledge of the time permitted. The treatments recommended were taken from the writings of Galen, an anatomist of the second century A.D., and from the Arabian writers. The emigration of Greek scholars to Western Europe during this period added much to dental and medical knowledge. Many of the contributors to the science of medicine also contributed much to dentistry—Vesalius, Fallopius, Eustachius, and Paré, to cite a few.

Pierre Fauchard (1690-1761) is considered to be the founder of modern scientific dentistry. His book *Le Chirurgien Dentiste* records the then-current technical aspects of dentistry to which he contributed greatly.

John Hunter (1728-1793), an English physician, also wrote extensively on dentistry. Two of his best-known works are *The Natural History of Human Teeth* and *A Practical Treatise on Diseases of the Teeth.*

Dentistry in the United States had its beginnings in the latter part of the eighteenth century and was based on the dental knowledge of Western Europe. John Boher, an Englishman, was probably the first competent dentist to practice in this country. Another was John Greenwood, who was dentist to George Washington.

Dental education in the United States had its beginning in Bainbridge, Ohio, under the guidance of John Harris, who was preceptor to his brother, Chapin B. Harris, and to James Taylor. These men later formed the first recognized colleges of dentistry in the United States.

The year 1839 is memorable in dental history for the establishment of a dental journal, the organization of a dental society, and the application for a charter to open a school for training dentists. In 1840 the Baltimore College of Dental Surgery, the first of its kind in the world, opened its doors.

Rapid technical advances in dentistry occurred after 1850. Among these were the discovery of vulcanite as a denture base material; the development of gold foil, gold inlays, and amalgam as filling materials; the invention of the dental engine or mechanical drill; and the use of X-ray films and local anesthesia. Two dentists, Dr. Horace Wells and Dr. W. G. T. Morton, first used general anesthesia in 1846 and are credited with being among the first to use a general anesthetic agent.

Under the leadership of Dr. G. V. Black (1836-1915), who next to Fauchard is the best-known figure in dentistry, dental education became truly scientific and professional. Dr. Black, who was Dean of the Dental School at Northwestern University in Chicago, performed brilliant research in anatomy and in the development of dental materials. He invented the foot-driven dental engine, and his classification of cavity preparations as well as many of the technical procedures he developed are still used today.

After World War II, new advances in dental equipment (notably the air rotor), materials, research, and methods of practice made it possible for the dentist to be much more productive than before.

PROFESSIONAL DENTAL EDUCATION

The length of predental training varies from two to four years. A very few exceptional students are admitted after only two years. About 30% of all incoming students have completed three years of undergraduate study and the rest have completed four years; nearly all students in this group have baccalaureate degrees. Many colleges have an arts-dentistry program in which the enrolled students attend

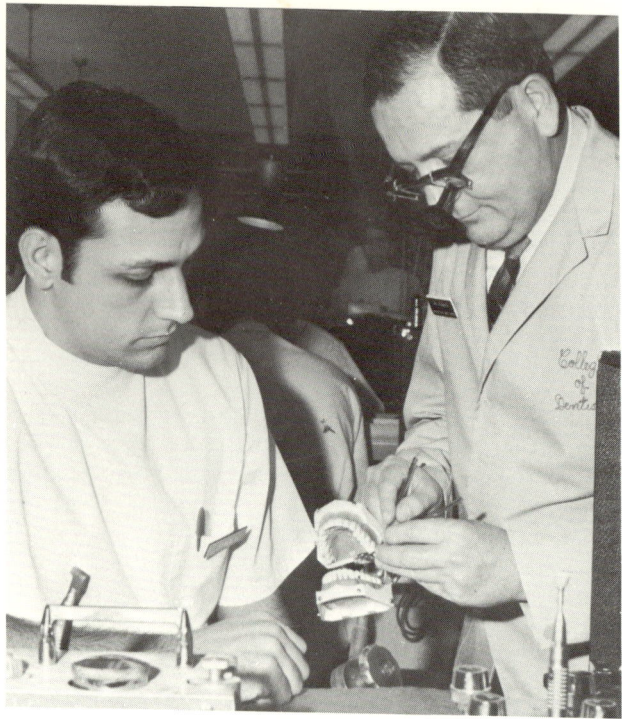

Fig. 3. Models of jaws and teeth are used in preclinical study to give students practice in instrument position and techniques.

a college of liberal arts for three years and earn a baccalaureate degree at the end of their first year in dentistry. Participation in this program makes it possible to earn two degrees in seven years. Predental students are encouraged to enroll in an arts-dentistry curriculum if it is available and are often given preference in admissions selection.

Required predental courses are kept at a minimum. These include such areas as the following:
1. English composition and literature
2. Biology, including zoology
3. General chemistry, including qualitative analysis
4. Organic chemistry with laboratory
5. Physics with laboratory

It is usually recommended that predental students pursue a broad educational program that includes the social sciences and humanities rather than overemphasize the basic sciences, as many of these are covered in the professional curriculum.

The objective of dental education is to train a student to be knowledgeable and competent in basic sciences, dental laboratory procedures, clinical dentistry, practice management, and social and preventive dentistry. This is much to accomplish in four academic years; consequently, the program is rigorous and difficult, challenging and demanding. (See Fig. 3.)

Because of the nature of the dental curriculum and the physical limitations on the numbers of new students who can be accepted into dental schools, competition for admission is very keen. All students are required to take a dental admissions test given by the Council on Education of the American Dental Association (ADA) at specific times at various testing centers. Admissions are based on predental academic performance, dental admission test scores, basic science grades, and a personal interview.

During the third academic year of the professional curriculum, students are eligible to take the first half of the written examination offered by the National Board of Dental Examiners of the Council on Dental Education of the ADA. Toward the end of the final year, students can take the second part of the examination. In addition, they must pass a clinical examination given by the state dental board of the state in which they desire to practice. On successful completion of this examination, they are permitted to practice only in that state. However, in some areas, regional examinations offer dentists who qualify a license to practice in each of several cooperating states.

SUPPORTING PROFESSIONALS

Most graduate dentists are engaged in private practice. In this situation a dentist or group of dentists has the responsibility for directing the activities of the office. The physical arrangement and facilities vary with each office, but the trend is toward multiple operating rooms and several auxiliary personnel such as dental hygienists, dental assistants, dental technologists, receptionists, and office secretaries. The dentist who utilizes these additional personnel can be much more productive and provide better service to patients than the dentist who conducts a one-person practice with little or no auxiliary help.

Recent changes in dental practice acts in many states now permit qualified dental hygienists and assistants to perform certain dental procedures that until now have been restricted to licensed dentists. These changes have resulted in increased productivity and efficiency in dental practices.

Training programs for dental hygienists are available at the college level. These professionals are skilled technicians and they may function as teachers in dental health education programs as well. They are becoming increasingly important in reducing dental disease. For the prospective hygienist who plans to work primarily in a private office, there are two-year professional training programs available, some of which award an associate degree. The profession of dental hygiene is discussed in greater detail in Chapter 2.

For dental laboratory technicians there are vocational school programs at the post–high school level as well as on-the-job training in a dental laboratory. Enrollment in an approved training program provides one year of formal training and a second year of supervised training in a commercial laboratory and is an effective preparation for this career. The tasks of dental laboratory technicians include making and repairing such dental restorations as dentures, inlays, crowns, and bridges. Their objectives are to promote better health, greater comfort, and improved appearance, and they always work from the prescription of a licensed dentist. Salaries for the experienced laboratory technician range from $8,000 to $14,000 annually.

A third type of auxiliary personnel is the dental assistant, who may be employed by an individual dentist or by a group of two or more practitioners. There are increasing employment opportunities for assistants in clinics, hospitals, and other health agencies. Dental assistants are responsible for greeting patients and preparing them for examination, treatment, or surgery. They sterilize instruments, mix fillings, prepare solutions, and help the dentist to practice his skills. The present trend in the profession is to utilize the assistants as part of the dental operating team in a system known as four-handed dentistry. In this capacity dental assistants perform in a manner similar to that of the surgical technician in the medical operating room. In smaller office situations dental assistants may also be responsible for such clerical tasks as making appointments, ordering supplies, sending out statements, keeping patient records, and answering the telephone. Many dentists are willing to select a likely applicant and provide on-the-job training. However, some dental schools, colleges, and junior colleges are offering training for dental assistants. Some programs offer an associate degree. Salaries for these workers range from $6,000 to $10,000 per year, depending on community salary standards, extent of training, and amount of experience.

FUTURE TRENDS IN DENTAL PRACTICE

The emphasis in modern dental practice is increasingly being placed on the prevention of dental disease and the maintenance of oral health. With modern dental knowledge and procedures, it is possible to maintain the entire dentition in good health for a lifetime. There is also growing interest in and concern for the social aspects of dentistry. The goal is comprehensive dental care for all people. There is now such a large backlog of patients with extensive dental problems that it is necessary for the dentist to spend much of his time in the treatment of dental diseases. The mode of dental practice has gradually been changing from individual dental practice to groups of dentists with the same specialty or groups with diverse specialties. Such groups result in increased efficiency. With these changes and currently available preventive measures such as fluoridation, dietary control, preventive treatment by the dentist, and adequate home care, it should be possible to vastly improve the oral health of our citizens.

CAREERS IN DENTISTRY

There are approximately 105,500 licensed dentists in the United States. About 9,100 are on the staffs of federal agencies (Air Force, Army, Navy, Public Health Service, Veterans Administration, Civil Service). Approximately 10,286 are engaged in dental education and research. The remainder are engaged in private practice. There are approximately 4,250 new graduates each year. When retirement and death of members of the profession are taken into account, it is evident that the profession is not likely to be overcrowded in the forseeable future.

Many graduate dentists continue their educational training and become qualified in one of the eight recognized specialties of dentistry.

Endodontics	Treatment of diseases of the internal soft tissues of the teeth
Oral pathology	Diagnosis of diseases or abnormalities of the oral cavity and associated structures
Oral surgery	Treatment of diseases or abnormalities of the oral cavity and associated structures
Orthodontics	Treatment of malocclusion and facial deformities
Pedodontics	Treatment of dental diseases in children
Periodontics	Treatment of diseases of the supporting structures of the teeth
Prosthodontics	Restoration of occlusion by replacement of missing teeth
Dental public health	Concern with dental epidemiology, biostatistics, and dental public health measures

With the exception of oral surgery, which is a three-year, hospital-based program, these specialties require from eighteen months to two years of additional training.

The income of most dentists is well above average. Few dentists become wealthy, but most enjoy a very comfortable life. The 1973 *Survey of Dental Practices* shows that the mean net income of all independent dentists for 1972 was $35,698. There is also a certain degree of prestige and respect afforded those dentists who are ethical in practice and have a genuine concern for their patients. According to a 1971 survey by Rotter and Stein in the *Journal of Applied Psychology,* dentistry was ranked third in a listing of twenty selected occupations by the public in terms of trustworthiness, competence, and altruism.

At the present time the energies of the dental profession are directed toward more sophisticated methods of practice, better delivery of dental services, prevention of dental diseases, and the community and social aspects of dentistry.

PERSONAL QUALIFICATIONS

The profession of dentistry is not suitable for everyone. Prospective dental students must have a good background in the basic sciences and the liberal arts. They must be industrious, intelligent, well motivated, and have a high degree of manual skill and artistic ability. They must have a concern for their fellow man and enjoy working with people. They must be competent at business and office management and should have analytical minds and the ability to work well independently. Among the most important attributes are a good character and high moral and ethical standards. It is wise for students who are seriously considering becoming dentists to learn as much as possible about the profession by attending career programs, reading, and visiting dental offices and dental schools. This insight should help them to determine whether dentistry is the profession they should pursue.

The practice of dentistry is confining, demanding, and conducive to tensions. It requires a great deal of self-discipline, but most dentists would consider the rewards well worth these disadvantages. For the person who qualifies to become a successful dentist there can be no more rewarding or satisfying profession.

REFERENCES

American dental directory 1974, Chicago, 1973, American Dental Association.

Annual report on dental auxiliary education 1973-1974, Chicago, 1974, Council on Dental Education, American Dental Association.

Annual report on dental education 1973-1974, Chicago, 1974, Council on Dental Education, American Dental Association.

Dalton, V. B.: Genesis of dental education, Columbus, Ohio, 1946, Spahr & Glenn.

Directory of dental educators 1973-1974, Chicago, 1973, American Association of Dental Schools.

Guerini, V.: A history of dentistry, ed. 1, Philadelphia, 1909, Lea & Febiger.

Lufkin, A. W.: A history of dentistry, ed. 2, Philadelphia, 1948, Lea & Febiger.

Prinz, H.: Dental chronology, ed. 1, Philadelphia, 1945, Lea & Febiger.

Rotter, J. B., and Stein, D. K.: Public attitude toward the trustworthiness and altruism of twenty selected occupations, Journal of Applied Social Psychology **1:**343, 1971.

Survey of dental practices 1973, Chicago, 1973, Bureau of Economic Research, American Dental Association.

PROFESSIONAL ORGANIZATION WHERE FURTHER INFORMATION CAN BE OBTAINED

American Dental Association
211 East Chicago Avenue
Chicago, Illinois 60611

Chapter 4
Dietetics
Burness G. Wenberg

Altering a person's nutritional status may affect physical condition, performance, personality, disposition, appearance, and life-span. New discoveries are constantly being made in the fields of medicine and nutrition. New and better methods and procedures for preparing and serving food appear almost daily, and new food products on the market have become almost commonplace. As a result, the profession of dietetics continues to change, grow, and expand to serve people better.

The dietitian is committed to improving human nutrition, advancing the science of dietetics and nutrition, and promoting education in these and allied areas. Food is the tool that the dietitian uses in illustrating and promoting good nutrition. Dietitians work with people of all ages in a variety of institutional and agency settings. (See Fig. 4.) Hospitals and health care facilities claim the greatest number of dietitians. They are also found in elementary and secondary school, college, and university food services. Others may be employed in business and industry. Teaching at the college level and research in food and nutrition are additional careers for dietitians. Many of the new and developing health maintenance organizations have dietitians on their staffs. For those persons interested in working with food and people, a variety of opportunities are available.

HOW DID THE PROFESSION DEVELOP?

Although the profession of dietetics is relatively young, its background reaches into antiquity. The Ebers papyrus, written a thousand years before Hippocrates, contained what may be the first recorded diet prescription. The famous French scientist Lavoisier made a revolutionary contribution to nutrition in 1794 by making laboratory determinations of the end results of digestive activities. For opening the door to scientific research in this field, he is accepted as the father of nutrition.

Continuing inquiry in this century has produced methods that make it possible to measure energy transformation in the body, to determine the exact nutritive values of food materials, and to determine the roles of proteins, minerals, vitamins, and other nutrients in the functioning of the body. Formerly dietitians were associated with the feeding of sick persons and worked almost exclusively in hospitals. As the

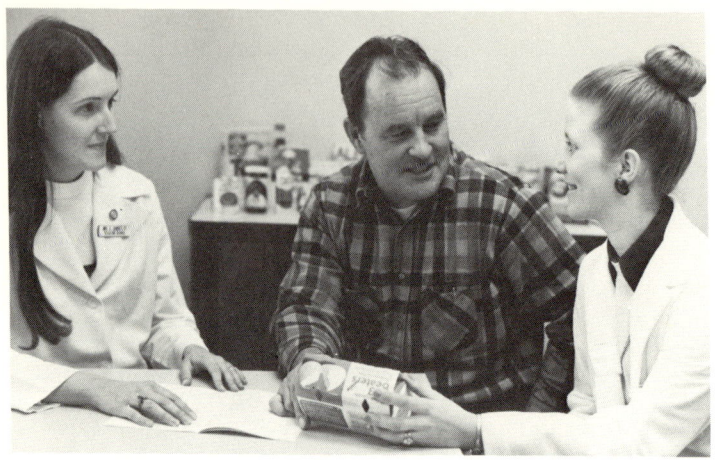

Fig. 4. Patients are encouraged to plan their own dietary program with the assistance of the dietitian and the student dietitian.

science of nutrition developed, dietitians have assumed the additional responsibility of applying research findings to the work of feeding groups of people.

The services of dietitians were in great demand during World War I, both in Europe with the armed forces and at home, where they faced the problem of feeding people in institutions despite the limitations imposed by food rationing and food shortages. Expressing a need to share their knowledge and seek better solutions to their problems, a small group of dietitians met in Cleveland, Ohio, in 1917 to organize the American Dietetic Association. The new organization's greatest impact may have resulted from its identification of educational requirements for curricula in dietetics and from its subsequent work with colleges, universities, and hospitals to implement these new standards.

Prior to 1917 there were a few "student dietitian" programs in hospitals. The applicants' qualifications ranged from a high school diploma to a college degree. By 1935 some sixty hospitals and institutions offered programs approved by the American Dietetic Association for the professional education of dietitians. Applicants to these programs were required to present a college degree, with successful completion of courses in foods, nutrition, and chemistry. As the number of dietitians as well as the quality of their training increased, both the profession and the professional organization gained in strength and stature. The professional dietitian achieved recognition as the person skilled in providing quality nutritional care to individuals and groups.

In 1970, with the financial support of the W. K. Kellogg Foundation, the American Dietetic Association charged a study commission with the responsibility for exploring all aspects of dietetic practice, education, and professional organization. The commission's report, published in 1972, included a review of current forces producing change in the field of health services. These findings led to the prediction that dietetic practice in the future would be altered in six ways: (1) there will be increased differentiation in the roles and functions of dietitians; (2) dietitians will become more specialized; (3) new and additional competencies will be required; (4) dietitians will increasingly delegate some of their present tasks and roles to other, less highly trained workers; (5) more dietitians will practice in association with other health professionals; and (6) a greater proportion of dietitians will be self-employed. Only the future will reveal the accuracy of these predictions.

WHAT PARTICULAR QUALITIES ARE NEEDED?

Young men and women should consider careers in dietetics if they (1) find studying the biological and behavioral sciences stimulating, (2) are interested in the nutritional, sociological, and psychological effects of foods on people, (3) enjoy working directly with people, and (4) gain personal satisfaction from using their knowledge to benefit mankind. The ability to be creative and innovative in the preparation and service of food is especially valuable to prospective dietitians. These individuals are entering a highly respected and relevant profession—a profession whose major concern is the welfare of humanity.

WHAT IS THE EDUCATIONAL PREPARATION?

Those who want to become professionally qualified dietitians will find that a variety of pathways lead to their goal. The professionally qualified dietitian has earned a bachelor's degree from an accredited college or university. In addition, successful completion of stated academic requirements and professional educational training, both approved by the American Dietetic Association, are required. The professional education component is available in a number of different methods and locations. Some are coordinated clinical-didactic undergraduate programs, while others are postbaccalaureate dietetic internships, dietetic traineeships, or graduate programs. Although some are specialized dietetic programs, the majority are more general. As different programs appeal to different students, they will be described separately.

High school

Preparation for a career in dietetics should begin in high school. College preparatory courses in chemistry, mathematics, biology, and the social sciences are highly recommended.

Academic requirements

A new plan for minimum academic requirements was adopted by the American Dietetic Association in 1972. Rather than specific courses, the requirements are stated in terms of competence to be acquired in specific areas. These include physical and biological sciences, behavioral and social sciences, professional sciences, and communication sciences. In addition, there are advanced competencies for general dietetics plus specializations in food service management and clinical and community dietetics. In presenting a dietetic curriculum, an accredited college or university selects and/or develops courses that include the stated competencies. These requirements may be incorporated into the curriculum of an undergraduate coordinated dietetic program or into a curriculum that serves as preparation for a postbaccalaureate professional education program.

Professional education programs

Coordinated undergraduate programs. Established in 1962, the coordinated undergraduate dietetic program is a formalized baccalaureate educational program in dietetics sponsored by an accredited college or university and accredited by the American Dietetic Association. The curriculum is designed to coordinate didactic and supervised clinical experiences to meet the qualifications for practice in the profession of dietetics. This type of program was first offered at The Ohio State University, and now an increasing number of colleges and universities throughout the United States are either offering or planning to offer such a curriculum. A list of currently accredited programs is published annually by the American Dietetic Association. Those who successfully complete such programs are recommended for membership in the American Dietetic Association concurrently with the awarding of the bachelor's degree.

Clinical or field experience is usually introduced in the junior year and increases in depth and scope with each succeeding term. Some programs focus on general dietetics, while others have a food service management, clinical, or community dietetics emphasis. Only those colleges and universities that have access to facilities adequate to provide the curriculum's clinical or field experience can offer this more specialized type of program. The undergraduate coordinated programs have the advantage of orienting students to the typical clinical or field experience setting for the practice of dietetics early in their educational experience.

Dietetic internships. The dietetic internship is a formalized postbaccalaureate educational program in dietetics sponsored and conducted by an organization and approved by the American Dietetic Association. The curriculum of the program is designed to provide didactic and supervised clinical experience to meet the qualifications for practice in dietetics. The Association annually publishes a listing of currently approved internship programs.

These internships provide an opportunity for the dietetic intern to practice in depth the principles of nutritional care and food service management learned in college. Under the guidance of an experienced staff and faculty, dietetic interns add to their basic knowledge and develop their own professional behavioral style. The dietetic internship has been traditionally viewed as the "fifth year," but since early 1970 there have been many innovations in both existing and developing dietetic internships. Programs that are now offered vary in length from six to eight, nine, ten, twelve, fifteen, and eighteen months. Approved dietetic internships are offered in a variety of institutions: hospitals, nutrition clinics, industrial food services, school food services, state institutions, and colleges and universities. Basically, nutritional care in a hospital or an outpatient clinic and food service management in a variety of food service settings are emphasized. Successful completion of a dietetic internship qualifies the graduate for membership in the American Dietetic Association.

Dietetic traineeships. The approved, preplanned experience program was the forerunner of the dietetic traineeship. First offered in 1973, the traineeship is an individualized, postbaccalaureate educational program in dietetics sponsored by an organization and approved by the American Dietetic Association. Each program is designed to provide didactic and supervised clinical experience to meet the qualifications for practice in the profession of dietetics.

In accordance with the concept of an individualized program, a traineeship program is developed and arranged between a qualified candidate and the registered dietitians in an organization willing to sponsor such a program. Programs must be at least twelve months in length and may focus on general dietetics or clinical or food service management. Successful completion of a dietetic traineeship qualifies the graduate for membership in the American Dietetic Association. Published essentials of a dietetic traineeship may be obtained from the Association.

Graduate study. Membership in the American Dietetic Association can also be obtained by earning a master's degree and experience or a doctoral degree. Recipients of a master's degree in foods, nutrition, food service management, dietetic education, or public health nutrition must satisfactorily complete the equivalent of six months of work experience under the supervision of a professionally qualified dietitian. The recipient of a doctoral degree in any in these areas of specialization is eligible for membership. As graduate programs do not require prior approval, documentation of achievement in the curriculum and endorsement by at least one professionally trained dietitian are required when application for membership in the association is made.

WHO ARE REGISTERED DIETITIANS?

The registered dietitian is an American Dietetic Association dietitian who has successfully completed the examination for registration and meets continuing education requirements. An American Dietetic

Association dietitian is described as a specialist educated for a profession that is responsible for the nutritional care of individuals and groups. This care includes the application of the science and art of human nutrition in helping people to select and obtain food for the primary purpose of nourishing their bodies in health or disease throughout the life cycle. This work may be accomplished through single or combined functions, in food service systems management, in extending knowledge of food and nutrition principles, in teaching the application of these principles according to individual situations, or in dietary counseling.

The concept of professional registration was adopted by the members of the association in 1969, and registration is voluntary for members. Each member is free to participate or to abstain, and continuing membership in the association remains entirely unaffected by participation or nonparticipation in the plan. The abbreviation R.D. stands for registered dietitian and is a trademark of the association that registered dietitians may use. Registration was adopted with the goal of maintaining and enhancing the standards of the profession and its individual practitioners.

WHERE DO DIETITIANS WORK?

There are many areas of service available to the dietitian. Many choose to work in hospitals or clinics, while some prefer the atmosphere of nursing homes or extended care facilities. Others find research, community health services, food service management, or teaching especially rewarding. Dietitians may find that they are the only member of their profession employed in a given setting, or they may be a member of a dietetic staff that ranges in size from two to as many as the twenty-five or thirty professionals found in large teaching hospitals.

Clinical dietitians employed in hospitals or extended care facilities work closely with physicians and other health care personnel in selecting appropriate diets and in providing dietary care. Those working in a nutrition clinic or with groups involved in community health projects will be associated with physicians, social workers, and public health nurses. They may participate in individual counseling and group education. The clinical dietitian may find it helpful or even necessary to visit people in their homes to assist them in the wise purchase, storage, and preparation of foods.

What specifically might the clinical dietitian's job be? Miss Jones is employed by the nutrition services department of a large medical center. She is one of a staff of eight dietitians and is responsible to Miss Webster, the head dietitian of the Service. Miss Jones is assigned to a ninety-patient medical unit, and she works with all of the health professionals on that unit. Her working day usually runs from 7:30 A.M. to 4:30 P.M. She begins her day by checking with the dietetic technician on new admissions, diet changes, and planned discharges of patients. Today Miss Jones must meet with three patients who are going home by 10:00 A.M. She promised to see them before they left in case they had any additional questions about the low-salt diets they are to follow at home. There are also ten new patients to be seen. Miss Jones' task is to assess their need for nutrition counseling and make plans for any further dietary counseling. Between 9:00 and 11:00 A.M. she works with those patients in need of dietary counseling.

As this is Tuesday, it is the day of the chief of staff's weekly luncheon conference with medical students, interns, and residents. Miss Jones participates in these conferences of patient presentations and contributes her knowledge to the identification and solution of their nutritional problems. From 2:00 to 3:00 P.M. she participates in daily class activities that the unit presents for all of the patients with diabetes. Today Miss Jones has the class on diet. As soon as she returns from class, the head nurse calls her to report difficulty with the 2:30 P.M. tube feeding for one of the patients. Miss Jones checks immediately and discovers that the recipe she developed had not been followed. To resolve the problem, Miss Jones supervises its preparation so she may be certain that the patient receives what he should and that the food service worker understands how to follow the new recipe. That was Tuesday! Wednesday will bring some of the same activities, but there will be a whole new set of challenges as well.

The administrative or food service management dietitian is responsible for planning menus, ordering the required food, and organizing and supervising the food service workers who prepare and serve food to the clientele. The clientele may be children in school lunch programs, students who participate in college and university food service programs, employees in industrial cafeterias, customers in commercial cafeterias, or patients in hospitals or extended care facilities. In fact, food service management dietitians can be involved wherever food is served to groups of people.

Let us look at the typical day of a dietitian in a school lunch program to gain a better understanding of the work of a food service management dietitian. Miss Smith is the only dietitian employed in the New School District, which operates five elementary schools and a junior and senior high school. The total enrollment is 2,000 students. The kitchen is located in the senior high school, and food prepared there is transported by truck to the other schools. Miss Smith has a staff of three dietetic technicians and twelve food service workers. When she arrives at 8:00 A.M., Miss Smith checks with the dietetic technicians to ensure that the assigned workers are on duty and that all the food needed for the day is available. Her calendar for today includes a meeting with one of the fifth-grade classes at 10:00 A.M. to assist the teacher in presenting a nutrition unit. Miss Smith must also check on a complaint that food is cold when it arrives at the junior high school at 11:30 A.M. She meets at 1:30 P.M. with one of the elementary school PTAs to finalize plans for a spaghetti supper and must attend the superintendent's meeting with all the school district's principals at 3:00 P.M. to discuss the defeat of the operating tax levy at the previous day's election.

Today is Thursday, and therefore the orders for all of next week's deliveries of meat and fresh vegetables and fruit must be placed. As you can see, this food service management dietitian must be able to work with people, must enjoy working with food, and must be ready to seek solutions to a variety of problems.

These are just two examples of the dietitian's world of work. Nutrition research, college teaching, and many other opportunities are available to the qualified dietitian.

WHAT IS THE NEED FOR DIETITIANS?

Dietitians are in great demand today, and this demand will continue to increase for many years to come. Presently there are 25,000 members of the American Dietetic Association, approximately 500 of whom are men. The percentage of men entering the field is increasing each year.

It is estimated that 56,000 qualified dietitians will be needed by 1980. In order to satisfy this need, approximately 5,000 persons should be entering the field each year through 1980, but in fact approximately 1,000 join the profession each year.

Because the supply is not meeting the demand, job opportunities available to those entering the field are many and varied. Salaries continue to increase, and fringe benefits become more attractive. The American Dietetic Association has recommended a minimum annual salary of $11,000 for the association dietitian who has just completed educational requirements and is entering the practice of dietetics. The association's recommended minimum salary for the beginning registered dietitian is $12,000.

WHO ARE THE SUPPORTING PROFESSIONALS?

Departments of dietetics in hospitals, extended care facilities, schools, and other institutions employ people who are qualified to assist dietitians in specific areas of food service management and nutritional care. These supporting professionals play an important role in the dietetic or food service department. Their major objective is to contribute to the nutritional welfare of the patient or client. Their duties may vary according to the size and type of institution for which they work, but they are always interesting, satisfying, and rewarding.

Dietetic technicians

The dietetic technician is a technically skilled person who has successfully completed an associate degree program that meets the educational standards established by the American Dietetic Association. As of June, 1975, the successful graduate of such a program is eligible for associate membership in the American Dietetic Association. Graduates of other dietetic technician programs are required to document equivalent education and experience. The technician, who works under the guidance of a registered or American Dietetic Association dietitian, has responsibilities in assigned areas in food service management, in teaching foods and nutrition principles, and in dietary counseling. To better understand the role of the technician, the following tasks are a sampling of what might be included in a job description. Dietetic technicians plan menus based on established guidelines; maintain and improve standards of sanitation, safety, and security; select, schedule, and conduct orientation and in-service education programs for personnel; obtain, evaluate, and utilize information on dietary history in planning nutritional care; calculate nutrient intake and dietary patterns; and utilize appropriate verbal and written communication and public relations skills, inter- and intradepartmentally.

Dietetic assistants

The dietetic assistant is a skilled person who has successfully completed a high school education or the equivalent and a dietetic assistant's program that meets the standards established by the American Dietetic Association. The assistant, working under the guidance of a registered or American Dietetic Association dietitian or a dietetic technician, has responsibility in assigned areas for food service to individuals and groups. Typically dietetic assistants are responsible for assisting in the standardization of recipes and testing of new products; instructing personnel in the use, care and maintenance of equipment; assisting in implementing cost control procedures; recommending improvements in facilities and equipment; processing dietary orders, menus, and other directives related to patient care; and helping patients to select menus. Like dietetic technicians, dietetic assistants may be employed in food service departments of health care facilities, educational institutions, or industry.

SUMMARY

Dietetics is one of the well-established health professions that is concerned with both sick and well persons. Food is the tool the dietitian uses to promote nutrition by assisting in the maintenance of good health and in the prevention and treatment of disease. Prospective dietetic students may choose from a variety of educational programs and, depending on their interests and abilities, may select one of a number of available areas for an in-depth study of dietetics. As food—nutritious food—is essential to life, there will always be a need for dietitians.

REFERENCES

Allied health manpower, 1950-80, Publication No. 263, Sec. 21, Washington, D.C., 1970, Department of Health, Education, and Welfare, United States Public Health Service.

Position paper on recommended salaries and employment practices for members of the American Dietetic Association, Journal of the American Dietetic Association **67:**139, 1975.

The profession of dietetics, approved programs 1974-1975, Chicago, 1974, American Dietetic Association. Titles, definitions, and responsibilities for the profession of dietetics 1974.

SUGGESTED READINGS

Kinsinger, R. E., editor: Health technicians, Chicago, 1970, J. G. Ferguson Publishing Co.

Report of the committee to develop a glossary on terminology for the association and profession, Journal of the American Dietetic Association **64:**661, 1974.

The profession of dietetics. The report of the study commission of dietetics, Chicago, 1972, American Dietetic Association.

PROFESSIONAL ORGANIZATION WHERE FURTHER INFORMATION CAN BE OBTAINED

American Dietetic Association
430 North Michigan Avenue
Chicago, Illinois 60611

Chapter 5
Extracorporeal circulation technology
James P. Dearing

Extracorporeal circulation technology is a new addition to the allied health professions. It was conceived and developed during the past decade through the efforts of many people from several disciplines. Medicine and engineering combined skills to develop this new technology in response to a need that had been apparent since the late 1950s.

Extracorporeal circulation technologists play a vital role in caring for patients undergoing heart surgery. They also provide circulatory support for a failing heart or lungs, remove toxic products from the blood stream by means of the artificial kidney, deliver chemotherapeutic agents to the cancer patient, and make possible a variety of diagnostic procedures. All of these techniques put the patient's circulatory system in direct continuity with instrumentation either for monitoring purposes or for the removal, processing, and subsequent return of the patient's blood to his own circulatory system.

PROFESSIONAL DEVELOPMENT

Since the first successful elective open heart operation supported by cardiopulmonary bypass was performed in 1953, there has been a remarkable growth in extracorporeal (outside the body) circulation technology. In 1974 there were more than 100,000 such operations performed in more than 1,000 institutions in which a heart/lung machine was available. (See Fig. 5.) Concurrent with the first open heart procedures, hemodialysis (removal of wastes from the blood via the artificial kidney) became an accepted treatment for patients suffering from kidney failure. (See Fig. 6.) There are now more than 200 hemodialysis centers registered with the Kidney Disease Control Program of the United States Public Health Service.

During the early developmental days of extracorporeal circulation technology, the devices used were physician developed and physician operated. Gradually this responsibility has changed hands, as physicians recognized that it was an inefficient use of their time and that their medical training did not encompass the engineering skills required for continuing development of the technology.

The first nonphysician operators of these devices were specially trained nurses, bioengineers, and physiologists. These highly educated

32 Introduction to health professions

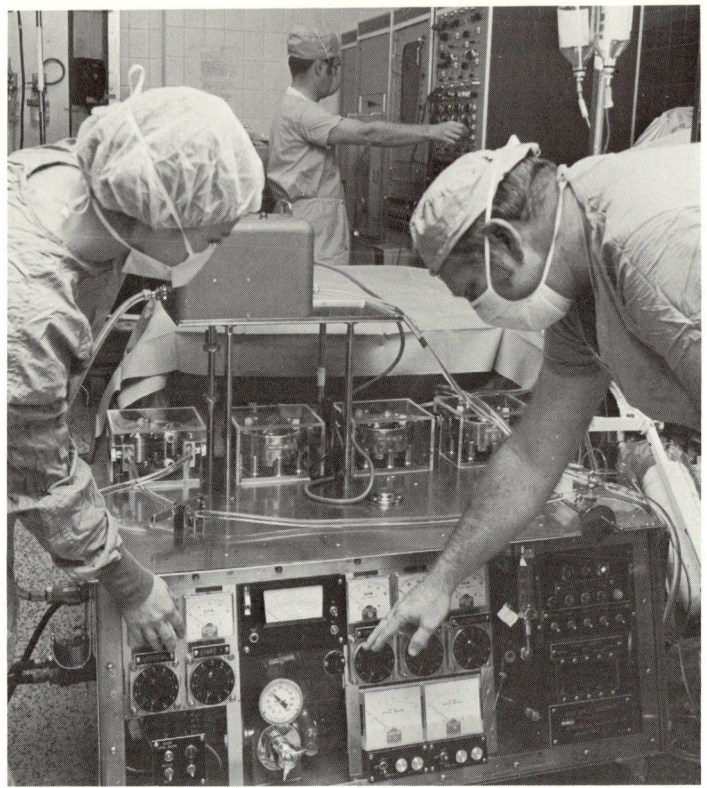

Fig. 5. Preparation of the heart-lung machine that is used to provide circulatory support for patients undergoing open heart surgery requires meticulous attention to detail.

specialists soon found that the demands on their time were too great, and therefore the responsibility was further relegated to a corps of competent technicians. During the past several years it has become evident that the knowledge of these technicians has become diluted because they have been trained primarily by other technicians rather than by the physicians, bioengineers, and physiologists who trained the first technicians in this field. At present the backgrounds and training of technicians are extremely varied.

Because of the lack of well-defined criteria for training and qualification, a concentrated effort was launched in the late 1960s to identify and define the practitioners in this technology as a new allied health profession. The approach was two-fold: first, to develop a curriculum and standards for the education of these specialists and second, to qualify the existing technologists.

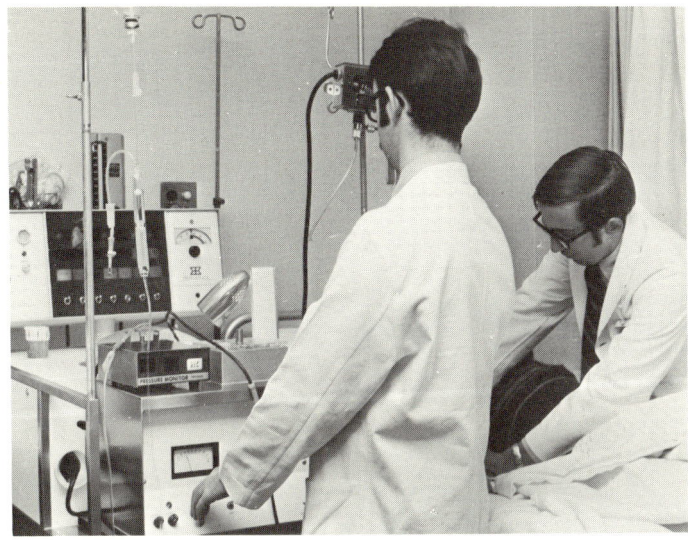

Fig. 6. Circulation technology students set up and operate the instrumentation for the hemodialysis of a patient.

The School of Allied Medical Professions at The Ohio State University committed itself in the late 1960s to the development of a curriculum in extracorporeal circulation technology. The objectives of this program were to provide a cadre of highly competent technologists and to provide a model for other educational programs.

In order to define that body of knowledge unique to the profession of extracorporeal circulation technology, a committee representing several disciplines—medicine, surgery, nursing, engineering, education, and biology—met to establish the curricular objectives for this new program. Once this body of knowledge was delineated, methods of presentation and evaluation were developed and converted into course descriptions, syllabi, and lesson plans. A permanent faculty representing both the biological and engineering aspects of the program was recruited and supplemented by guest faculty from nursing, medicine, education, pharmacology, veterinary medicine, and physiology. This effort has been duplicated at several other institutions, and a variety of training programs are now in operation and undergoing evaluation. Some of these programs limit their offering to only one aspect of extracorporeal circulation technology such as hemodialysis, while others encompass the entire field.

Concurrent with the development of educational programs, an effort to identify and qualify the technologists already practicing in the field was launched through an examination program developed by the technical society representing most of the practitioners.

EDUCATIONAL REQUIREMENTS

In November of 1974 the American Society of Extracorporeal Technology established minimum standards for training programs in extracorporeal circulation technology. These criteria were established to encompass all of the training programs currently in existence. The criteria establish the administrative and faculty requirements for schools and define minimal curricular requirements. The elements of the required curriculum are:

Course area	Clock hours
Anatomy and pathology	36
Physiology	36
Pharmacology	36
Extracorporeal circulation technology	48

In addition to the didactic requirements there is a clinical experience requirement of a minimum of twenty unassisted clinical cases. This requirement may be met in an internship program in an approved clinical institution if the institution offering the program does not have the clinical case load. On completion of an approved program, graduates must be employed in this field for six months before they are eligible to take the certification examination.

The examinations were developed through the process of examining only those technologists that meet two requirements: a minimum of two years in the field and a minimum of 100 unsupervised clinical cases. It was felt that these technologists had stood the test of time and thus their skills level could be used to standardize the certification examination for new entrants in the field. To date approximately 700 technologists have been certified through this examination process.

CAREER OPPORTUNITIES

Due to the rapid growth of medical practice that has required the support of extracorporeal circulation, technologists find an open career market. Although most technologists are employed by large medical centers, some have developed their own private groups that provide service to several hospitals on a fee-for-service basis. Others have gone into practice with a medical group. With the rapid growth of clinic dialysis, many career opportunities exist in privately operated clinics that specialize in ambulatory patient hemodialysis. Finally, there is a demand for well-educated and trained personnel in industry.

The salary range is broad. Annual starting salaries for new graduates range between $8,000 and $15,000. This wide range reflects both the differences among training programs and the types of jobs available. The higher salaries are commanded by those graduates with extensive knowledge in all areas of the technology and who are given the responsibility of developing and coordinating efforts in all of these areas.

SUMMARY

Extracorporeal circulation technology is a new, exciting, and demanding profession that offers the practitioner a challenging career at the leading edge of medical and technological advance. The profession deals with the use of artificial organs to sustain life and with the development of new and better techniques for performing this task. The emergence of this technology into a profession offers an enticing opportunity for those who enjoy applying engineering principles to the solution of biological problems.

SUGGESTED READINGS

Cromwell, L.: Biomedical instrumentation and measurement, Englewood Cliffs, N.J., 1973, Prentice Hall.

Norman, J. C.: Cardiac surgery, ed. 2, New York, 1972, Appleton-Century-Crofts.

Rushmer, R. F.: Cardiovascular dynamics, ed. 3, Philadelphia, 1973, W. B. Saunders Co.

PROFESSIONAL ORGANIZATION WHERE FURTHER INFORMATION CAN BE OBTAINED

American Society of Extracorporeal Technology
6352 Oakton Street
Morton Grove, Illinois 60053

Chapter 6
Health education
Mary Alice Beetham

Health education is a relatively new profession. In March of 1973 the report of the Joint Committee on Health Education Terminology* officially defined health education as "a process with intellectual, psychological, and social dimensions relating to activities which increase the abilities of people to make informed decisions affecting their personal, family, and community well being. This process, based on scientific principles, facilitates learning and behavioral change in both health personnel and consumers, including children and youth."

Health educators are identified professionally as school health, public health, or community health educators. The trend has been to recruit school and community health educators at the baccalaureate level. *School health* educators have received a teaching certificate and are respected members of public school systems with expertise in an identifiable subject area. Opportunities for employment outside the classroom encouraged the revision of teacher training programs so that professional preparation became available for *community health* educators. The *public health* educator is predominantly educated at a school of public health and earns a master's degree. Public health educators have long been respected members of the public health team in agencies where the team concept is revered.

SCOPE OF HEALTH EDUCATION

In R. M. Titmuss' terms, health education is a social service activity that is intended for the well-being of the population. In the terms of the Joint Economic Committee of the United States Congress, health education contributes to the development of human resources. Scott Simonds, Professor of Health Education at the University of Michigan School of Public Health, states that individual behaviors have a great deal to do with health outcomes and that a considerable reduction in morbidity and mortality rates could be achieved by informed and "health-activated" citizens. To compound existing societal problems, a

---

*This committee consists of representatives of the American Academy of Pediatrics; American Association of Health, Physical Education, and Recreation; American College Health Association; American Public Health Association; American School Health Association; and Society of Public Health Education, Inc.

recent study by Smith et al. showed that 5% of all television time in a metropolitan area was allocated to transmitting inaccurate or misleading health information. During the 1974 Federal Focus on Health Education Conference in Atlanta, Dr. Charles Edwards, Assistant Secretary for Health, United States Department of Health, Education, and Welfare, called for health education "not for education's sake but for its impact on total health." He cited lowered morbidity and mortality rates as a measure of health education. Successful programs are demonstrated by "each and every segment of society working toward a common objective measured in human terms" with each individual possessing a "sense of responsibility for (his) own health, as well as that of the community."

At the present time, according to the Report of the President's Committee on Health Education, there are 25,000 professional health educators in the nation—persons with bachelor's, master's, or doctoral degrees in either school or community health education.

School health education reaches 55 million children in the United States (one fourth of the entire population). The first ten years of life are cited by many experts as being the most crucial in terms of physical and psychological development, yet school health education is often not given much emphasis in the curriculum until the senior high school level. Hopefully, new federal comprehensive health education legislation will be forthcoming. Meanwhile, groups such as parent-teacher associations and medical auxiliaries are actively championing comprehensive health education. The Ohio State Planning Committee for Health Education did pioneering work in a legislative committee to achieve cooperation between official state agencies and health-related organizations in order to move health education from a paper priority to an action priority.

Community health education reaches out to the adult population primarily through programs at places of business (40% of the population is employed) and through television and other public media. A recent achievement in television programming is "Feeling Good" (The Children's Television Workshop), an adaptation of "Sesame Street" in the area of adult health, dedicated to the importance of health maintenance and prevention of illness.

PERSONAL QUALIFICATIONS

A school health educator needs basically the same qualifications as any other certified teacher, because these educators are concerned mainly with classroom teaching. Socrates said, "Example is not *one* method of teaching but the *only* method." A health teacher should embody positive physical, mental, and social health. Identification and imagery are very important, particularly to the elementary student. Love and respect for self and others is paramount. A sound informational base is required, but a teacher who enjoys teaching and who believes fundamentally that learning can be fun is assured of success. Skill as a facilitator of learning is a professional asset.

A community health/public health educator also must have a sound informational base but needs more preparation in communications and group process skills, since much education will be accomplished through committee teamwork and community organization. The educational focus is on the nonschool community. The public health educator holds the philosophy that if you teach one person who in turn teaches another, the "multiplier effect" is seen, whether the teaching is through intermediaries, personal instruction, or mass media. A good community health educator must be interested in working with people. An extroverted personality is helpful but not essential. The positive health image is essential because a community health educator is in public view. It is difficult to "sell" trimness when one is fat or the dangers of smoking while one is lighting a cigarette.

EDUCATIONAL PREPARATION

The school health educator receives a bachelor's degree in education and meets the basic requirements for any teacher certification program. This includes a student teaching requirement. Preparation in health education may be as a major or minor field.

The community health educator is a graduate of a bachelor's degree program that may or may not include a period of student teaching. The usual substitution for student teaching is supervised field work. The program may be based in a college of education or school of allied health professions.

The public health educator is a master's degree recipient (M.P.H. or M.S.P.H.) from a school of public health. A list of accredited schools may be obtained from the American Public Health Association (APHA). Also, universities such as the University of Tennessee that are accredited in community health education have a master's degree program following a school health education program as well as an APHA-accredited master of science degree. Doctoral degrees are offered in both health education and public health education.

CAREER OPPORTUNITIES

Because health educators are not licensed, there is a tremendous variety of employment possibilities and personal emphases. School health educators are usually found in public school settings; with graduate degrees, they may teach in colleges or universities. Many voluntary health agencies utilize persons experienced in this discipline as program directors. Official agencies such as city and state health departments add them to their teams of health educators within the agency and also in program areas.

Community health educators are sought by official and voluntary agencies and recently have joined the staffs of health planning programs, neighborhood health centers, community mental health centers, hospitals, clinics, industries, and other community projects. Public health educators are able to satisfy requirements for consultative positions (federal, state, and local), administrative positions in health-related fields, and occasionally collegiate appointments in addition to opportunities in community health. Growing numbers of public health educators work as "patient health educators" in the provision of health care services. As health maintenance organizations gain visibility and as the criteria are established for health education as a benefit reimbursable through health insurance programs, this role is becoming more established. Hospitals are now being encouraged to expand their services to include patient education. Some form of national health insurance is imminent, and prevention of illness through health education will be stressed. There are four basic criteria for judging the effectiveness of any national health program or facility: (1) accessibility, (2) availability, (3) acceptability, (4) accountability. Without health education, accountability would not be possible within our economic restrictions. Health educators will help to ensure the acceptability of health care programs through the application of communicating and listening skills.

SUMMARY

Health education is a profession that bridges the gap between health information (what one knows) and health practices (what one does). It must start at the level of the learner. The responsibility of individuals for their own health has always been of paramount importance to the school health educator, although collectively these same individuals are the primary targets of community-wide health education.

Health educators must encourage the productive effort of health education by all—the health team (governmental, voluntary, and private agencies) and the general public joining hands, so to speak. Many prominent health educators believe that optimal physical, mental, and social health is possible for all. The potential for all children to be born healthy and wanted depends on health education that reaches the parents of our nation's children before conception and therefore contributes to a better quality of life. Attitudes and behavior reflect values and decision making. A sense of responsibility for individual and community health is essential.

REFERENCES

Joint Economic Committee, United States Congress, Subcommittee on Economic Progress: Federal programs for the development of human resources, Washington, D.C., 1966, United States Government Printing Office.

Proceedings of the federal focus on health education conference, Washington, D.C., 1974, United States Department of Health, Education and Welfare.

Report of the President's Committee on Health Education, Health Services, and Mental Health Administration, Washington, D.C., 1973, United States Government Printing Office.

Smith, F. A., et al.: Health information during a week of television, New England Journal of Medicine **286:** 516, 1972.

Titmuss, R. M.: Commitment to welfare, New York, 1968, Pantheon Books, Inc.

PROFESSIONAL ORGANIZATIONS WHERE FURTHER INFORMATION CAN BE OBTAINED

Society for Public Health Education, Inc.
655 Sutter Street
San Francisco, California 94102

American Public Health Association, Public Health Education Section
1015 Eighteenth Street, N.W.
Washington, D.C. 20036

American Association for Health, Physical Education, and Recreation
1201 Sixteenth Street, N.W.
Washington, D.C. 20036

American School Health Association
P. O. Box 708
Kent, Ohio 44240

Chapter 7

Hospital and health services administration

Barbara McCool

Health services administrators have the responsibility of managing the complex organization of a hospital, public health agency, health maintenance organization, or other health-related facility. Their main role is to marshal and coordinate the resources necessary for the delivery of health care.

Usually the health care administrator is directly responsible to a board of trustees, a group of civic-minded community leaders who determine broad policies and objectives. The administrator directs the day-to-day activities of the institution and assumes a major role in planning and promoting the development of health care services. (See Fig. 7.) In larger institutions this may involve supervising and coordinating the activities of more than thirty highly specialized departments that perform administrative, professional, or maintenance and operational services.

Health care administrators act to ensure that the health care facility operates efficiently as a unit; they see that necessary facilities, equipment, and services are available; they help to coordinate the development of educational programs for nurses, physicians, technologists, and other personnel; and they oversee the facility's contributions to preventive medicine and to improving the health of the people the facility serves. Besides providing the optimum internal environment, the administrator represents the health institution in the community, in the state through membership in state associations, and nationally through participation in the work of associations that represent such special interest groups as the American Hospital Association, the American Public Health Association, and the Association of Mental Health Administrators.

HISTORY OF THE PROFESSION

The institutionalization of health care in the United States began in 1752 when Benjamin Franklin and Dr. Thomas Bond established the Pennsylvania Hospital in Philadelphia. The early hospitals were viewed as boardinghouses for the poor and terminally ill. As advances in medical science were made, the hospital became the focal point of

42 Introduction to health professions

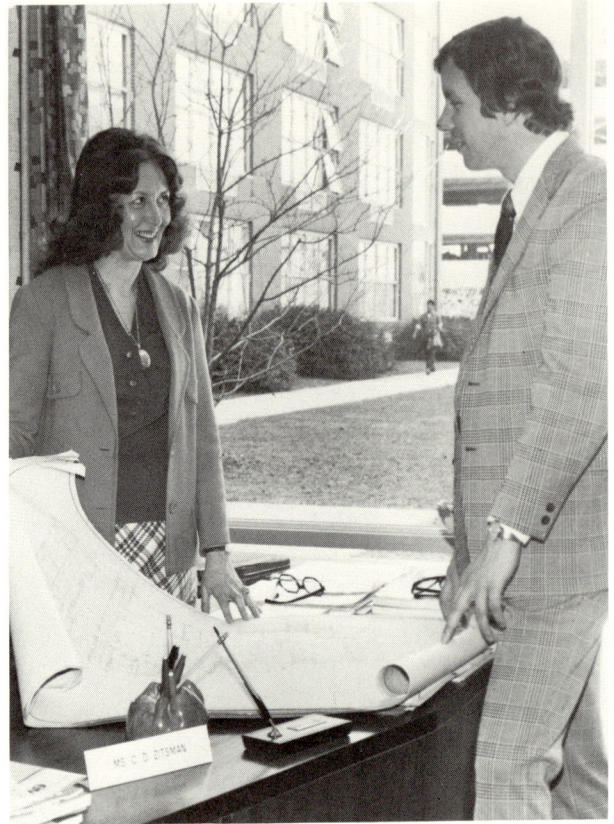

Fig. 7. Hospital administrators plan future health services.

care and continued to grow in importance and complexity. There are approximately 7,000 hospitals in the United States today.

Parallel to the development of the modern hospital has been the evolution of the profession of hospital and health services administration. The early hospitals were managed on a part-time basis by a physician or nurse whose primary responsibility was to act as the custodian of property and equipment. As medical care became more complex and as governmental, legislative, and community factors grew in influence, administrative responsibilities also grew.

Hospital and health services administration became a profession with the formation of the American College of Hospital Administrators in 1933 and the beginnings of graduate education in health services administration in 1934. The goal of the American College of Hospital

Administrators was to develop standards of performance and education. Concomitantly, the first graduate program in hospital and health services administration was started in 1934 at the University of Chicago. Other graduate programs were developed to prepare professional administrators, and today there are approximately seventy-six operational programs.

EDUCATIONAL PREPARATION

Preparation for a career in hospital and health services administration takes place at the graduate level. After earning a bachelor's degree, students should apply to the graduate program of their choice.

Programs in hospital and health services administration provide students with an in-depth familiarity with modern management concepts and with the community, organizational, technical, political, and socioeconomic environments within which these concepts must be applied.

The curricula of the various programs that offer graduate study reflect the particular emphasis of the university department of which they are a part, such as medicine, business, or public policy. Some programs require two academic years on campus with summer work experience in a health facility, while others require one year on campus in academic work and a second year in an administrative residency at a health services institution.

On completion of their formal education, new graduates usually start their professional careers as administrative assistants in a hospital, insurance firm, public health agency, or health maintenance organization.

Undergraduate programs are a new development in education for hospital and health services administration. At the present time, thirty-five institutions offer a baccalaureate degree for persons who wish to become middle managers in large health institutions or administrators of extended care facilities and other health agencies of similar size.

PERSONAL QUALITIES NEEDED

A future health care administrator should possess (1) a commitment to serving others, (2) above-average intelligence, (3) the ability to get along with many different kinds of people, (4) the ability to work under pressure, and (5) adequate physical and emotional stamina.

RELATED PROFESSIONALS

The hospital and health services administrator works with physicians, community and business leaders, government officials, and a wide variety of health professionals to organize and coordinate health care delivery for a defined population. Within the health care institution the administrator creates an environment in which highly skilled health professionals can apply their knowledge and skills to the care of the patient.

• • •

A profile of one day in the life of a hospital administrator illustrates the challenges facing today's health administrator. Richard Cramer is the administrator of Northfield Community Hospital, a 400-bed, general acute care institution operated by a nonprofit corporation in a midwestern city with a population of 500,000. It offers medical, surgical, pediatric, obstetrical, and psychiatric care programs, has modern diagnostic and therapeutic facilities, and cooperates with other hospitals in the area in operating a comprehensive outpatient clinic. It is fully accredited by the Joint Commission on Accreditation of Hospitals and sponsors several medical and allied health educational programs. Mr. Cramer has been the administrator of Northfield for three years. He is active in the American College of Hospital Administrators, serves as a delegate to the American Hospital Association, and is President of the State Hospital Association. He has three assistant administrators, all of whom are active in the civic life of the community.

8:00 Mr. Cramer arrives at the hospital parking lot and is stopped by Dr. Kenneth Stone, Chief of the Medical Staff. Dr. Stone arranges a meeting with Mr. Cramer for 1:30 that afternoon to review the applications of physicians who have applied for medical staff privileges.

8:15 As he approaches the entrance to the hospital, Mr. Cramer meets Mrs. Evans, a member of the hospital's Board of Trustees. Mr. Evans is currently a patient at Northfield, and Mr. Cramer is pleased to learn that Mr. Evans is recuperating from his surgery and will be going home in a few days.

8:25 When Mr. Cramer arrives at his office, his secretary, Miss Rolfe, hands him his appointment schedule for the day, a folder of correspondence, and a list of several phone calls that must be returned. Mr. Cramer glances quickly through his mail, which includes a letter from the Blue Cross Association concerning a revised reimbursement schedule, several thank you notes from patients who have been discharged from the hospital, a letter from the hospital's attorney explaining the institution's legal position in a pending liability case, bids from contractors for construction of a new facility, a letter of resignation from a department head, and confirmation of his reservation for the upcoming annual meeting of the American College of Hospital Administrators.

8:30 Mr. Cramer's three assistants and the Director of Nursing Services arrive for their daily meeting. Mrs. Smiley presents the patient census for the day and reports on events that occurred on the night shift and on the condition of critical patients. Mr. Pace distributes copies of the pharmacy reorganization plans that will be presented at the meeting of department heads later in the day. He also announces that he will be representing the hospital at the certificate of need hearing with the comprehensive health planning agency. Mr. Brooks reports that the parking lot construction will be slowed down by a delay in the delivery of entrance gates and that representatives of the housekeeping employees' union have approached him about negotiations for a new union contract. Mr. Parks mentions that he and Dr. Summerfield will be leaving the next day to recruit interns and residents for the following year. Mr. Cramer announces that the revised wage and salary program will be discussed at an administration meeting to be held the following day, when a decision will be made about implementation. During a discussion of plans for a new coronary unit, the hospital's architect arrives with drawings to be submitted to the Board of Trustees for approval. During the meeting, Miss Rolfe is busy answering telephone calls and arranging appointments. The meeting ends abruptly as the administrator is summoned to the emergency room, where the town's mayor has just been brought in following an automobile accident. Mr. Cramer instructs Miss Rolfe concerning notification of the press.

10:00   The President of the Board of Trustees arrives to discuss the agenda for the Board meeting to be held that evening.
11:30   Mr. Cramer addresses a luncheon meeting of the Kiwanis Club on the subject of national health insurance.
1:30   Dr. Stone arrives to review applications for medical staff privileges. The physician wants Mr. Cramer's recommendations prior to a meeting of the Credentials Committee that is scheduled for the following week. A problem that has arisen in the Anesthesiology Department is discussed and resolved.
3:00   Mr. Cramer attends the meeting of department heads and gives a report on the new management training program.
4:00   In a meeting with the hospital Comptroller, the Director of Nursing, and the Personnel Director, Mr. Cramer discusses the Nursing Service budget.
6:00   Mr. Cramer attends a dinner meeting of the Executive Committee of the Board of Trustees and discusses long-range development plans to be presented later at a meeting of the full Board.
10:00   Following the Executive Committee meeting, Mr. Cramer returns briefly to the hospital to check on the mayor's condition. He is relieved to find him resting comfortably and to learn that his injuries are not serious.

NEED FOR HOSPITAL ADMINISTRATORS

The rapidly expanding demand for comprehensive health care has intensified the need for competent hospital and health care administrators. This has become one of the critical issues facing the American health care system today, and the shortage of administrators will become more severe with the increased emphasis on extended care facilities, community mental health centers, expanded general hospitals, and area-wide planning agencies. Newly graduated hospital administrators may earn from $10,000 to $12,000 annually. Depending on the size of the facility, experience, and competence, an administrator may eventually earn from $25,000 to $30,000 a year.

SUMMARY

Today's health care delivery system is undergoing critical reexamination. Hospital and health services administrators are restructuring health care delivery systems so that all segments of the population may have equal access to comprehensive health services at costs lower than at present. The health care arena is characterized by change in virtually every area of its operation. In this dynamic milieu the hospital and health services administrator is faced with changing financial requirements, quality control systems, new mergers, government regulations, and other pending changes in national health policy. Those responding effectively to these challenges receive both the material rewards of high status and salaries and the many intangible rewards associated with human service.

SUGGESTED READINGS

Education for health administration. Report of the Commission on Education for Health Administration, Ann Arbor, 1974, University of Michigan Health Administration Press.

Hospital administrators, SRA Occupational Brief No. 235, Chicago, 1972, Science Research Associates, Inc.

Kirk, W. R.: Your career in hospital administration, Chicago, 1972, American College of Hospital Administrators Press.

United States Department of Labor, Bureau of Labor Statistics: Hospital administrators, Washington, D.C., 1970, United States Government Printing Office.

PROFESSIONAL ORGANIZATIONS WHERE FURTHER INFORMATION CAN BE OBTAINED

American College of Hospital Administrators
840 North Lake Shore Drive
Chicago, Illinois 60611

The Association of University Programs in Health Administration
#1 Dupont Circle, N.W.
Suite 420
Washington, D.C. 20036

Chapter 8
Medical communications
John E. Burke

The field of medical communications has evolved in the last several years as a result of a strong interdisciplinary challenge. As the demand for greater numbers of better-trained health professionals and improved health information systems became more urgent, there was clearly a need for communications specialists and researchers with a variety of skills. As communications technologies became more sophisticated, their applications in clinical and educational areas were explored by professionals with widely varying backgrounds in media, education, engineering, health, and the computer, behavioral, and social sciences.

Increases in population and information, together with advances in technology, brought communications specialists into a new relationship with many health professionals. (See Fig. 8.) This relationship, which began as consultation, has grown broader as communication problems have been recognized in every sector of biomedical education and indeed at every level of health care delivery. What has emerged is a new type of health professional with special background and skills in communication and an understanding of the needs and priorities of the health professions.

The importance of communication in the health care system has increased dramatically in recent years. The effective dissemination of health information is critical in controlling disease. Practitioners as well as scientists need current research information, teachers need better ways of transmitting an increasing volume of knowledge to larger numbers of students, and the consumers of health services need to know what services are available and where and how they may be obtained. Most important, the public needs to know how to stay well.

In order that patient care may be improved, the health care system must strengthen itself internally. Here again, communication is increasingly significant. Members of the health care team must learn better methods of communicating with each other as well as with their patients. They must understand their respective roles, cooperate in the development of hospital and public health information systems, and work together to find solutions to the many communications problems

Much of the material for this chapter is based on the chapter prepared by Kathryn Schoen for the first edition of this book.

48   *Introduction to health professions*

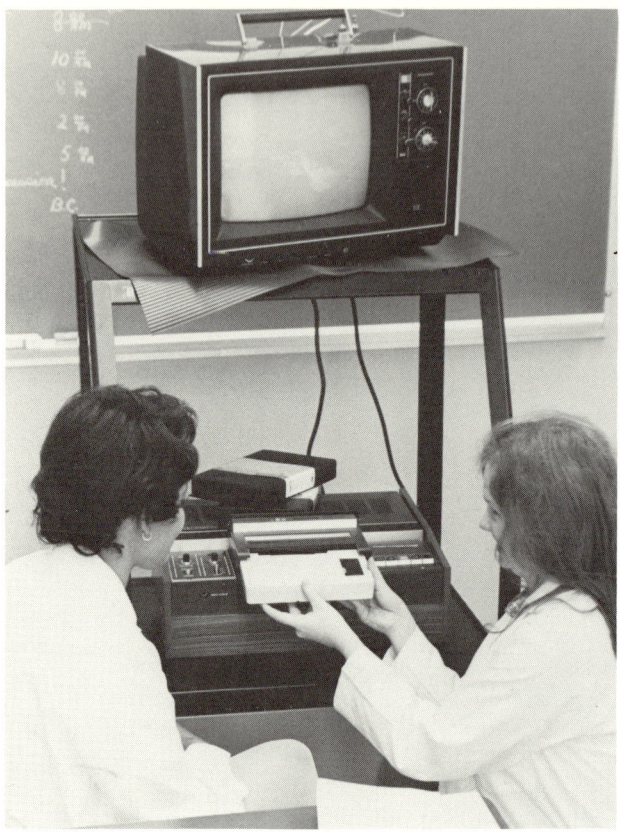

Fig. 8. Medical communications specialists work with many different health professionals in a variety of settings to improve communication effectiveness.

peculiar to the health professions. As Walker has pointed out, if the health care system is to continue to increase its efficiency, it must learn to cope with the new patterns and methods of communication.

Although a global definition of biomedical communication is still being refined, its basic components are clear. Whether it be in formal education in the health sciences, postgraduate education, in-service training, public information, clinical support systems, or research and development, the role of medical communications is to improve information transfer, processing, retention, and utilization. This implies a knowledge of behavioral change in its many forms, especially as it affects the health care delivery system. Although many professionals with special communications skills can be found in the health sciences, few practitioners have been trained specifically for this aspect of their work. Those such as medical illustrators, biomedical photographers, and medical librarians, who have received special training, usually work in highly specialized areas and are rarely involved in solving communications problems outside their special areas of expertise. It is extremely difficult to find professionals trained in communications in the broader sense who also know the language and environment of the health sciences. Generalists as well as specialists are needed to solve the many complex communication problems in modern health care. Programs have therefore been developed to train the professional medical communicator.

HISTORICAL DEVELOPMENT

Communications media and concern for the communication process are not new to the health professions. Indeed, written communication combined with aural and visual reinforcement is as old as medical science itself. Examples include the writings of Hippocrates, the anatomical drawings of Leonardo da Vinci, and the functional operating theaters of the late nineteenth century that were designed for the effective "audiovisual" orientation of young surgeons. The most dramatic communications advances, however, have come in this century. Progress in electronic technology, photography, and other media forms, combined with a better understanding of human communication, has led to exciting experimentation in medical education and communication. New learning systems are being introduced into medical education in an effort to meet the challenge for more and better-trained health professionals. The quality of the presentation of content (the instructional message) and the choice of proper media (film, audio, television, computers, slides, etc.) are fast becoming an important part of the repertoire of every educator in the health professions. Microwave interconnection, satellite transmission, closed-circuit telemedicine, and computerized information systems are all examples of advanced technologies being used today to help solve health care problems in a complex society.

Before the more revolutionary advances in communications technology such as television and the computer, other media were used to improve medical education and clinical services. Books, drawings, models, specimens, audio tapes, films, etc. all continue to be important tools of the medical communications specialist. With the introduction of television in the 1940s, however, medical communications became a more significant force in both educational and clinical settings. The expense and complexity of television and later the computer prompted biomedical and communications professionals to share ideas regarding the use of these new media. In 1953 the Audiovisual Conference of Medical and Allied Sciences was organized to further audiovisual education. If these early efforts did not solve the communication problems in the health sciences, they at least brought them into focus.

The first training programs in biomedical communication, organized in the 1960s, emphasized the technological and managerial rather than the social and behavioral aspects of communication. The objective of these educational programs was to harness the new technologies for the improvement of medical education. Trainees were drawn from professional schools or doctoral programs and exposed to various types of media applications and management systems, principally in large medical centers. One such training program was initiated by the National Medical Audiovisual Center in cooperation with Tulane and other universities. Other programs were sponsored by the National Library of Medicine to prepare specialists to manage the automated and information storage and retrieval networks that have been designed to improve the flow of biomedical information. More recently, several other undergraduate, postbaccalaureate, and graduate programs have evolved in an attempt to meet the growing demand for communications specialists in the health sciences. The graduate programs in biomedical communication are generally more flexible than the undergraduate training programs, although most focus on the management of instructional technology systems. Most undergraduate programs have been more specialized, emphasizing such aspects as instructional media or biomedical photography.

THE OHIO STATE UNIVERSITY PROGRAM

The first broad communications program for the health areas at the undergraduate level was initiated at The Ohio State University in 1969. With its philosophical foundations in the behavioral and health sciences and the parent disciplines of communication and education, the medical communications program was developed in much the same way as baccalaureate degree programs in other allied health disciplines. The four-year curriculum leads to a bachelor of science degree. Developed with a five-year grant from the Bureau of Health Manpower Education, Division of Allied Health Manpower, the program was designed to prepare entry-level professionals whose knowledge of communication theory and biomedical science would be sufficiently broad to consider various types of communication-based problems in health areas and whose skills training would be sufficiently strong to provide an operational base from which to begin. With these objectives established, a problem-solving approach emerged as the foundation for the professional curriculum, which begins in the junior year. Prior to entering the professional curriculum, prospective medical communicators must meet basic university requirements in liberal arts and develop an interdisciplinary approach to communications theory and skills. The schedule in the preprofessional program provides maximum exposure to disciplines related to medical communications and includes courses in photography and cinematography, television and audiovisual production, communication theories and models, biology, psychology, and sociology.

Potential students are screened carefully by the faculty before admission, as student selection is an extremely critical determinant of program success. Students are selected on the basis of interest and performance during the first two years, with emphasis placed on aptitude and interest in the behavioral and communications sciences. Having been admitted to the program in their third year, students begin their orientation to health sciences communication. As allied health students, they interact with other health science students and professionals both in and out of class and begin to develop a "feeling for the field." The professional curriculum includes courses in communication, education, human anatomy, medical science, management and statistics, writing and editing, followed by more specialized courses in advanced media production in biomedical communication, design and evaluation of instructional systems, and biomedical computer systems application. Students attend special seminars in the psychosocial aspects of disease and in organizational development. The curriculum relies heavily on the resources of the College of Medicine and the medical center. This provides the student with the opportunity to gain "real world" experience while still in training in such areas as the Medical Audiovisual and Television Center, the Center for Continuing Medical Education, the Computer-Assisted Instruction Regional Education Network, the Nisonger Center for Mental Retardation, University Hospitals, and the Patient Education Network as well as other departments and divisions within the College of Medicine. Students have the opportunity for independent study in such areas as patient and health personnel interaction, medical language, mediated teaching and learning, and teleconsultation and diagnosis. They learn to select the media or means of communication most appropriate for their own designs. Working and studying in a medical environment provide the medical communications student with the opportunity to develop a strong professional identity and the confidence to relate to other health professionals as equals. These experiences are essential to the development of a stable biomedical communications curriculum at any level.

During the fourth year in the baccalaureate program, students are required to spend fifteen or more hours weekly during each of two quarters in "clinical" or field experiences. The students are assigned to "preceptors," or supervisors, who act as both teachers and models to the students. They may be assigned to such diverse areas as an inner-city health center, the Colleges of Veterinary Medicine or Dentistry, community hospitals, or the drug crisis center. Students have done part of their internship in the Information Offices of the National Institutes of Health, research centers, and volunteer organizations such as the American Lung Association and the American Heart Association. In the "clinics," students are required to focus their unique interdisciplinary background, media skills, and knowledge of the medical and behavioral sciences on problems and projects assigned by their preceptors. They are responsible for the total design, implementation, and evaluation of their projects subject to the same constraints of time, space, and money as any other staff professional. Students also meet in class to discuss their problems and progress. Many of the preceptors have faculty appointments in the Medical Communications Division and often serve as guest lecturers. Experience has shown that preceptor and internship programs are very valuable elements in the training of medical communicators.

Medical communications majors may continue their formal education at the graduate level. Building on knowledge and skills acquired at the undergraduate level, medical communicators may move from the role of generalist to that of specialist through graduate study. For example, a new interdisciplinary graduate program at The Ohio State University will train biomedical computer and information specialists. Students with an interest in computer and information science and undergraduate training in medical communications may focus on the many special applications of the computer in biomedical education, research, and information processing. A more flexible master's program in the School of Allied Medical Professions allows the medical communications graduate to pursue interests in research, education, or administration with an emphasis on biomedical communication.

GRADUATE MEDICAL COMMUNICATORS

The multidisciplinary nature of their profession requires medical communicators to be generalists. They must learn to work effectively with all types of health professionals and consumers of health care in a constantly changing environment with its incessant priorities. Thus medical communications graduates must be sensitive to change, work comfortably with it, and indeed, often serve as its agent. With respect to the celerity of change within the field as well as the environment in which it is developing, it is important that medical communications professionals avoid what Edgar Dale has referred to as "frozen perspectives," that is, inflexible definitions or attitudes in an emerging profession. They must be eclectics who are prepared to use many specialties to coordinate and improve communication and instruction in the health sciences. Their approach must be creative and dynamic, and they must be ready to change with the needs and priorities of the health care system. With their academic foundation firmly fixed in communication, education, and the health sciences, medical communicators should take an integrative, humanistic, and holistic approach to both clinical and educational problem solving. As process consultants, they must be sensitive to the human as well as the professional needs of their clients as they analyze, evaluate, organize, coordinate, and activate any new system or project. (See Fig. 9.)

Graduates of baccalaureate programs may serve as communications consultants or media specialists in large teaching hospitals or smaller

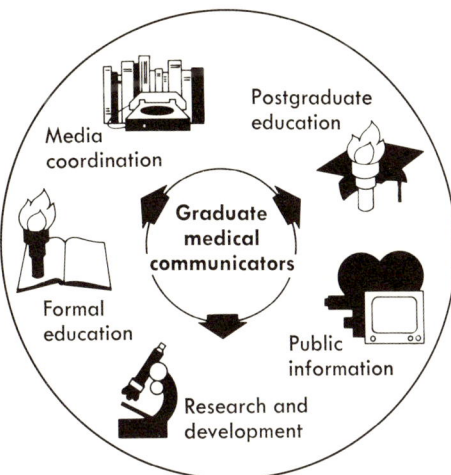

Fig. 9. Medical communications graduates work in a variety of areas in the health care environment.

community hospitals. They may coordinate educational media programs, participate in the design and implementation of communications research in the medical environment, or assist health agencies, professional organizations, and educators to communicate with either lay or professional audiences. They may assist in the planning and development of instructional aids or work in publishing or public relations. Whatever their role in the health care system, medical communicators continually evaluate all related communication efforts in order to improve their effectiveness. They are allied health professionals capable of conceptualizing and designing action-oriented programs to coordinate health needs, communication principles, media, and people.

Graduates of The Ohio State University program have accepted positions in health care centers such as the Cleveland Clinic, government settings such as the National Institutes of Health or the South Carolina Medical Television Network, teaching institutions such as the Columbia University School of Nursing, the University of Arizona Colleges of Medicine and Nursing, and the Indiana University College of Medicine, pharmaceutical firms, cancer research programs, computer centers, volunteer health organizations, and mental retardation centers. They have such titles as instructional resource specialist, instructional programmer, public relations specialist, coordinator of media services, hospital personnel director, director of training, and research assistant. It is interesting to note that of the members of the first two graduating classes, no two graduates accepted a position with the same title. Their unique interdisciplinary background prepares medical communicators for a wide variety of new and existing career opportunities in the health care system.

SUPPORTING PROFESSIONALS

The broad area of medical communications draws on the expertise of many contributing professionals and technical personnel to meet its goals and objectives. The graduate medical communicator relies on such specialists as medical photographers, medical librarians, educational developers and researchers, computer programmers, electronics engineers and technicians, and medical illustrators, the visual communicators of the health professions. These specialists must also be both versatile and exacting in their contributions to the field of medical communications.

The graduate medical communicator recognizes the importance of the many specialized contributors who help to meet the demand for improved communication services in the health field. The needs are too far-reaching and the goals are too important to work in isolation.

SUMMARY

Medical communications is concerned generally with facilitating the transfer of information for the improvement of health care, both directly and indirectly. Medical communicators, still fresh on the professional scene, use their unique interdisciplinary training in communications theory and media and their knowledge of the medical, social, and behavioral sciences to disseminate information for the improvement of patient care. They select and evaluate techniques to enhance biomedical education and to facilitate communication patterns in all areas of an increasingly complex health care system.

REFERENCES

Burke, J. E.: Medical communications as a health science discipline, Paper presented at the sixteenth annual meeting of the Health Science Communications Association, Denver, Colo., 1974.

Dale, E.: Personal communication, 1973.

Walker, H. L.: Communication and the American health care problem, Journal of Communication **23**:349, 1973.

PROFESSIONAL ORGANIZATIONS WHERE FURTHER INFORMATION CAN BE OBTAINED

Health Sciences Communications Association
P. O. Box 79
Millbrae, California 94030

Health Education Media Association
P. O. Box 5744
Bethesda, Maryland 20014

Chapter 9
Medical illustration
Mitzi Prosser and James R. Kreutzfeld

Medical illustrators are health professionals who design, illustrate and graphically represent biomedical facts, research data, surgical procedures, pathological studies, and anatomical plates. As an important member of the health care team, the illustrator works with physicians, research scientists, allied health professionals, and educators to visually record the constantly changing knowledge and skills of the ever-expanding medical profession.

HISTORY OF MEDICAL ILLUSTRATION

Medical illustration is as old as civilization, as indicated by the primitive anatomical drawings done on the walls of cave dwellings during the Stone Age. Leonardo da Vinci (1442-1519) made a lasting contribution to the science of anatomy. He combined curiosity, acute observation, and artistic talent to produce remarkable sketches that can still be used as teaching aids today.

During the 1500s there were several factors that influenced the growth of medical illustration. Woodblock carving was developed early in this period to help meet the demand for multiple copies of graphic art as well as written material. This led to the production of books, the first available mass-produced materials. Raffaello Santi's accurate depiction of the human body leads us to believe that his sketches were based on the direct observation, dissection, and investigation of cadavers. Jan Stephan Kalkar illustrated the anatomical works of Andreas Vesalius. Together they used woodcuts to produce the anatomical atlases *De Humani Corporis Fabrica*. From the expanded use of woodcuts to the development of copper engraving, the variety of visual aids used in educating people was increasing.

The introduction of the printing press, the invention of the process of lithography, and advances in photographic technique opened the way to more efficient methods of producing finished material. These processes were less expensive and required less time. The artists of the late eighteenth century were obviously influential in developing new and better methods for the reproduction of printed and graphic materials.

The early twentieth century saw the establishment of teaching centers where students could acquire the knowledge and skills necessary for a career in medical illustration. A leader in this area was Max Brödel (1870-1946), the man who has had perhaps the greatest influence in the field of medical illustration. Brödel established the first school of medical illustration at The Johns Hopkins University in 1910. He still remains the preeminent figure in medical illustration and has come to be known as the father of medical art.

EDUCATIONAL REQUIREMENTS

Students interested in the profession may choose one of seven recognized schools of medical illustration. There are variations in entrance requirements as well as in professional curricula. Some schools offer baccalaureate programs, while others offer programs leading to a graduate degree. For specific information concerning these programs, write to the individual schools or the Association of Medical Illustrators. Regardless of entrance requirements, students learn to adapt their artistic skills to the requirements of medical illustration and visual communication, acquiring at the same time a thorough background in the biological sciences.

Students in the professional programs develop skills in line, continuous tone, and color drawing techniques. Studies in biomedical photography, design, advertising, education, and management are an important part of the curriculum, as is training in the preparation of

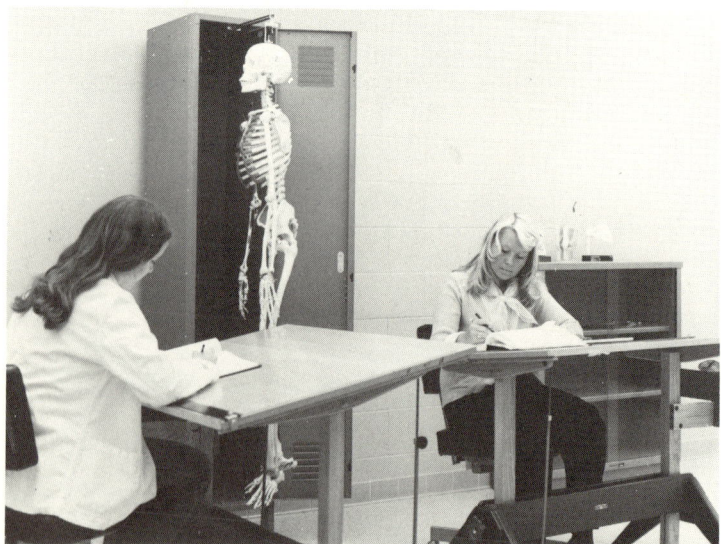

Fig. 10. Students perfect their drawing ability while learning various illustration techniques.

charts, graphs, and diagrams. Students are also required to take anatomy courses covering general and gross human anatomy, embryology, and histology. The acquired knowledge and developed skills are combined and integrated in the production of videotapes, films, and slide shows and in the preparation of exhibits, three-dimensional models, and prosthetics. (See Fig. 10.)

PROFESSIONAL MEDICAL ILLUSTRATION

Medical illustrators may receive assignments from a physician, researcher, or educator. For example, a surgeon may need a series of

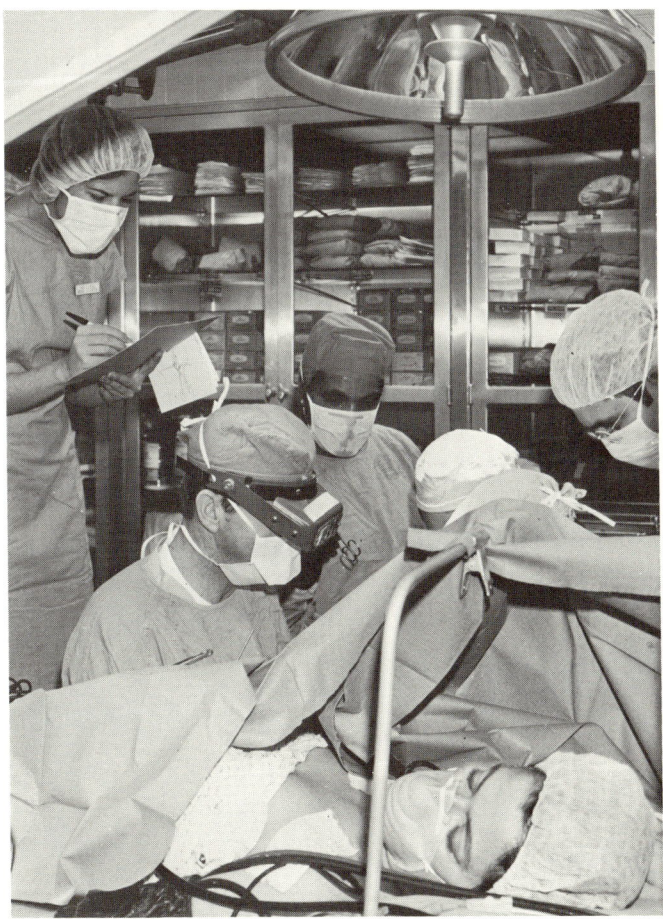

Fig. 11. Preliminary sketching of surgical procedures will result in a finished illustration to be included in a forthcoming textbook.

sketches of a particular operation. He calls on the medical illustrator, and together they review the operation before the scheduled surgery. During the operative procedure the medical illustrator may make sketches, take photographs, or both. (See Fig. 11.) Medical illustrators use these sketches or photographs and collaborate further with the surgeon in preparing the final renderings. Educational programs in medical illustration prepare students to execute finished illustrations of pertinent surgical, anatomical, and pathological aspects for use in medical textbooks, journals, and other media. These teaching aids are used not only for the education of medical students, interns, residents, attending staff, and allied health professionals but also for practitioners on a national and international level. They may also be used directly to educate patients regarding their own health care needs.

CAREER OPPORTUNITIES

Medical illustrators work in universities, medical or research hospitals and centers, scientific institutions, museums, pharmaceutical houses, publishing firms, and commercial art studios, or they may work on a free-lance basis for any of these agencies or for private physicians.

The beginning salaries in the field range from $8,500 to $12,000 annually, depending on the abilities and responsibilities of the illustrator and on the needs of the employer.

If medical illustrators wish to pursue their education at the graduate level, there are programs available that offer the opportunity to structure an interdisciplinary approach to an illustrator's specific problems and needs. Such a program may broaden concepts and strengthen skills in teaching, administration, communication, and research.

SUMMARY

Professional medical illustrators prepare visual materials for publications, exhibits, and teaching aids. The work requires artistic talent and scientific knowledge combined with accuracy, attention to minute detail, and technical versatility in each of the communications media. Medical illustrators use a wide variety of visual media such as drawing, painting, sculpture, and photography; the illustrations may be either realistic, diagrammatic, or representational. Some illustrators concentrate on work within one of the medical specialties. A medical illustrator is a highly trained artist who can conceive, design, illustrate, and produce visual material to inform and to educate members of the health professions as well as the entire community.

REFERENCES

Bethke, E. G.: Basic drawing for biology students, Springfield, Ill., 1969, Charles C Thomas, Publisher.

Clarke, C. D.: Illustration—its technique and application to the sciences, Baltimore, 1939, John D. Lucas Co., Publishers.

Vesalius, A., and Kalkar, J. S., De humani corporis fabrica, Cleveland, 1950, Cleveland World Publications.

SUGGESTED READINGS

McLarty, M. C.: Illustrating medicine and surgery, Baltimore, 1960, The Williams & Wilkins Co.

Price, F.: Medical illustration (do-it-yourself basis), Proc. Roy. Soc. Med. **62:**815, 1969.

Waters, L. B.: The mechanics of medical and dental visualization, Springfield, Ill., 1963, Charles C Thomas, Publisher.

Zollinger, R. M., and Howe, C. T.: The illustration of medical lectures, London, 1964, British Medical Association, vol. 14 (No. 3).

Zollinger, R. M., Pace, W., and Kienzle, G. J.: A practical outline for preparing medical talks and papers, New York, 1961, The Macmillan Co.

PROFESSIONAL ORGANIZATION WHERE FURTHER INFORMATION CAN BE OBTAINED

Association of Medical Illustrators
6650 Northwest Highway
Chicago, Illinois 60631

Chapter 10
Medical record administration
Melanie Moersch Pariser

> ... While the science of medical records has made great strides forward in recent years, the art of keeping records is as old as medicine.*

Medical record keeping is not a new concept. Information of a medical nature was recorded as far back as 25,000 B.C. Early cave drawings and relics relate the fact that ancient men of medicine understood the importance of keeping information on their medical achievements. Medical recordings in history served physicians of old as the medical record serves the physician of today. As medicine advanced throughout the ages, so did the need for better documentation and storage of medical information. It became more and more important for medical information to be written in a manner that would be usable for efficient patient care and for education. Early hospitals initially recorded patient information in log books; gradually they began to record all information in one place, a patient's medical record.

Techniques for recording, storing, and retrieving medical records were not really developed until the early twentieth century. At the turn of the century, medical schools and teaching hospitals recognized the need for better medical records and methods of keeping these records. Physicians pressed for standardization and quality in medical record keeping. The endeavors of these health professionals were instrumental in the development of the medical record profession.

Individuals responsible for the custodial care of medical records were brought together in 1928, and this group formed the American Medical Record Association. The objective of the new association was to strive for higher standards of patient care through better quality medical records. The medical record profession has continued to strive for this objective while growing to meet the demands of medicine and health care.

Today medical record administration is an allied health profession concerned with the design, implementation, and management of patient information systems. The profession combines a knowledge of both health care and business administration. Medical record administration

---

*From History of medical record science: from hieroglyphics to ... electronic data processing, Medical Record News **40:**20, 1969.

involves indirect contact with patients, for its emphasis is on handling of patient information rather than patients themselves. Patient information is recorded in medical records on every patient seen in a health care facility. The patient's record is the major component of a patient information system. The most important element of the medical record is the information recorded within it.

MEDICAL RECORDS

The medical record is the nucleus of patient information within a health care institution (See Fig. 12). All health care services involved in patient care funnel information to the medical record. The record is a story of the patient. It relates the who, what, where, when, and how of a patient's experience in a health care facility. Contents of a medical record include a history of the patient's illness and physical condition. The record reveals the physician's observations, findings, and orders. In addition, the medical record contains results of laboratory tests, X-ray findings, and nurses' notes. Pertinent reports such as those from surgery, pathology, and physical therapy are also included.

A patient information system and its major component, the medical

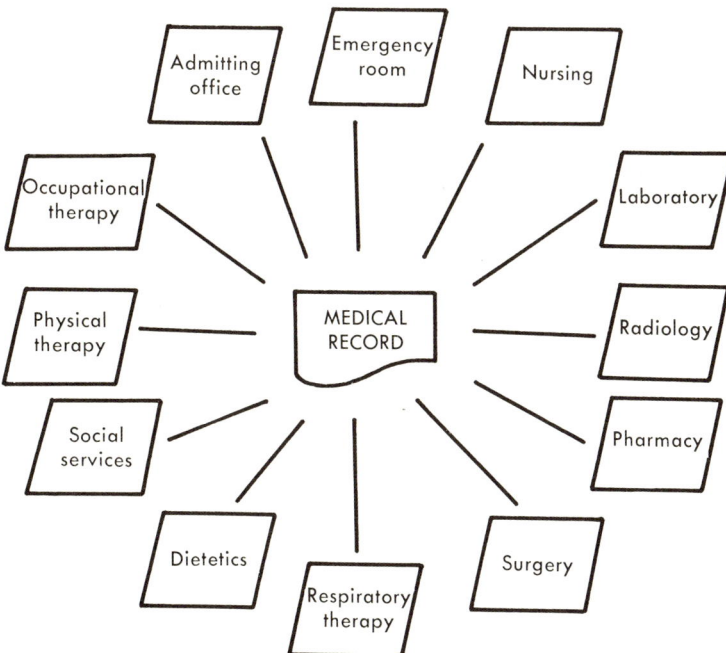

Fig. 12. The medical record is made up of information from all health care services.

record, is found in all types of health care facilities. Medical records are kept by hospitals, nursing homes, neighborhood health centers, mental health centers, ambulatory care centers, outpatient clinics, health maintenance organizations, rehabilitation centers, and doctors' offices. In some cases there are patient information systems in insurance companies and governmental agencies.

Medical records vary according to the type of health care facility involved. The medical record may be a hospital, psychiatric, or nursing home medical record. Ambulatory care centers and outpatient clinics often call the medical record a clinic record. Medical records of neighborhood health centers, mental health centers, health maintenance organizations, and doctors' offices are sometimes called health records.

The patient information system is the arrangement of methods for gathering, utilizing, storing, and retrieving medical information, for example, the different methods used to pull charts for a clinic, answer a subpoena for a court, or obtain information for research. Computer technology has been incorporated in patient information systems as more health professionals require access to records in order to ensure quality patient care. The computer offers a means of recording procedures and exchanging patient information at speeds unobtainable in the handwritten medical record.

PURPOSES OF MEDICAL RECORDS

All data concerning a patient are put into his record, including information on the patient's health problems, the treatments given, and results of therapy. Huffman has summarized the purposes of the medical record as follows: The medical record
1. Provides a means of communication between the physician and other professionals contributing to the patient's care
2. Serves as a basis for planning individual patient care
3. Furnishes documentary evidence of the course of the patient's illness and treatment during each hospital admission
4. Serves as a basis for analysis, study, and evaluation of the quality of care rendered to the patient
5. Assists in protecting the legal interests of the patient, hospital, and physician
6. Provides clinical data for use in research and education

The medical record is a *communication link* between all services within a health care facility. Physician, nurse, and allied health professional use the medical record to record their observations, findings, and treatments. They also use it to brief themselves on the patient's condition so that they know what has occurred since they last saw the patient. The medical record provides health professionals with an information base for planning patient care, not only for current problems but often for future care. For example, an unconscious woman who had previously been treated in the hospital for diabetes is brought to the

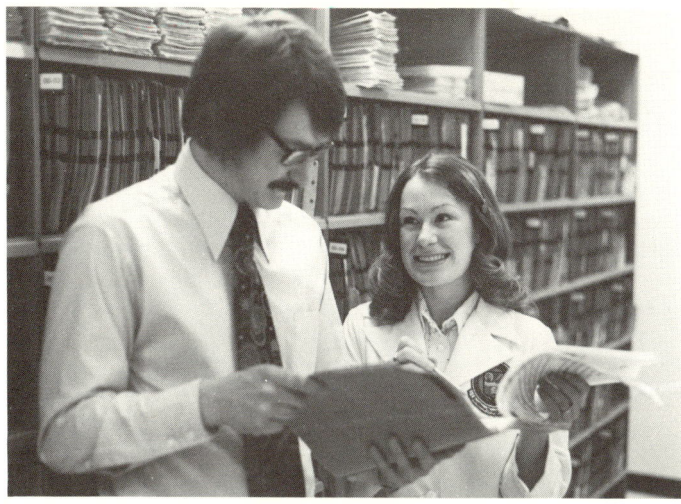

Fig. 13. A major responsibility of the medical record administrator is to assist medical personnel in record keeping, whether for patient care or for research.

hospital emergency room. The doctor thinks that she may be in a diabetic coma. He needs to know what treatment and medications the patient is already taking before he can prescribe for the current emergency. The medical record department is called, and the patient's record is brought to the doctor within minutes. The doctor is then able to refer to the medical record for the information he needs. (See Fig. 13.)

The quality of patient care is an important aspect of today's health care system. In order to ensure good care, health care institutions look inward at what happens in the facility. They do this by using the medical record. Because the medical record is a composite of all that happens to a patient, it becomes the health care institution's best device for *quality review*. The record is used to study and evaluate the quality of care rendered a patient. If properly documented, the medical record reveals the type of care a patient receives in a health care institution and is reviewed as evidence of services provided as well as quality of care given.

In legal cases the medical record is used as evidence of a patient's illness, treatment, and level of recovery. The record helps *protect the legal concerns* of the patient, physician, and health care facility. The patient may need to use his record to prove illness and disability in order to claim workmen's compensation. A physician may use a medical record to document his adequate treatment of a patient. The health care facility may turn to the record as proof that a nurse gave a correct medication. Whatever the legal concern, the patient, physician, or health care facility may consult the medical record for evidence of the care provided.

Medical records are a major source of data for use in *research and education*. Medical information in the record is essential for conducting retrospective and prospective research studies. It becomes a necessary tool in medical education. Medical researchers rely on medical records to provide them with necessary data for developing new techniques in the prevention and treatment of disease. The results of such research may be presented in medical or health journals and medical conferences or used as aids in educating health professionals. Records of research on a particular disease may assist in determining the need for a new treatment approach. Government agencies such as public health departments use medical records in determining incidence or trends in diseases and also to help discover community health needs. No matter what type of medical research and education takes place, the record serves as a basic source of medical data.

ROLE OF THE MEDICAL RECORD ADMINISTRATOR

Medical record administrators are the directors of medical record departments in health care facilities. They supervise and manage departmental employees in medical record keeping services. Medical record administrators coordinate departmental functions with the administrative, medical, ethical, and legal requirements of a health care facility and report directly to the health care facility administrator or to one of the assistant administrators. In some cases the medical record administrator is an assistant administrator of the health care facility.

Medical record administrators oversee the entire patient information system. They are aware of the informational needs of all health professionals and service departments within the health care facility. It is their responsibility to help these individuals to develop the best way of recording and also of retrieving patient information, using their knowledge of forms design and recording techniques to accomplish this. Medical record administrators must also be able to solve problems unique to specific situations, such as assisting a physician in reviewing medical records of patients with similar hereditary backgrounds or designing a method to help nurses review the kinds of nursing care given to patients with a specific disease.

At the departmental level, medical record administrators have complete administrative control. They are responsible for the design, implementation, and management of medical record keeping services and for the supervision of personnel. This includes departmental control of all budgetary, equipment, and supply needs. Medical record administrators must maintain a smooth and efficient means of gathering, storing, and retrieving all medical records.

Medical record administrators continually evaluate and, when necessary, improve procedures and forms utilized in departmental work. For example, a medical record administrator may investigate the current

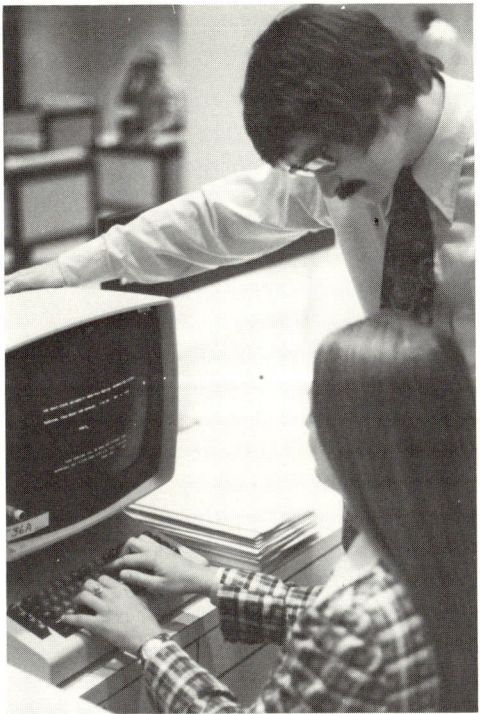

Fig. 14. The physician and medical record administrator refer to the computer terminal for needed medical information.

system of a manual patient index and decide that the manual index should be changed to a computerized system. Management skills would be used in assessing the old system as well as in planning and implementing the new. The new system may require that the administrator (1) design the format of information that will go on the computer, (2) assist the computer specialists in developing procedures for putting the information in the computer, (3) train personnel in the new procedures, and (4) develop a backup system for times when the computer is down. In the process of change, the medical record administrator acts as liaison between the people involved, such as data processing personnel and the medical staff. (See Fig. 14.)

In addition to overseeing departmental functions, the medical record administrator assists the medical staff of a health care facility in evaluating patient care and in reviewing medical and professional services within the facility by developing criteria and methods for evaluating medical records. The medical record administrator also aids the medical staff by explaining the requirements for completing medical records, carrying through governmental requirements for reporting care given to Medicare and Medicaid patients, and by acting as a resource person for all patient information needs.

The medical record administrator often acts as consultant and/or inservice educator for many departments in a health care facility, providing needed information for committees, offering courses in medical terminology to personnel from other departments such as the admitting office, or conducting classes to explain a new records procedure to those affected.

One of the most important responsibilities of the medical record administrator is protection of the confidentiality of patient information. The medical record administrator has a major responsibility for developing professional and ethical guidelines for the health care facility. These guidelines are used in developing policies and procedures for the release of patient information and in processing medical records for litigation. The medical record administrator is often looked to for guidance in handling records for legal purposes and in resolving problems of confidentiality.

Because of the growing need for experts to manage all types of health information within a community, medical record administrators often find employment outside hospital situations. Additional responsibilities emerge that reflect the changes in interagency information needs and in turn make changes in the job function of the medical record administrator.

The trend in medical record administration is toward increased dependence on computers for handling patient information. Medical record administrators already rely on computers for such departmental functions as patient indexing, scheduling patients, and requesting record retrieval for clinics, printing out doctors' incomplete medical records, abstracting medical data, computerizing the disease and operation index. Eventually patient information systems and individual medical records will be completely computerized. Medical record administrators will have to expand their knowledge and responsibilities according to the advances in computer technology. In the future, they will most assuredly be known as health information coordinators.

PROGRAMS IN MEDICAL RECORD ADMINISTRATION

To become a registered record administrator (R.R.A.), an individual must successfully complete an approved program in medical record administration and pass the national registration examination of the American Medical Record Association (AMRA). There are approximately forty approved programs of medical record administration in colleges and universities throughout the United States. These programs must be approved by the American Medical Association's Council on Medical Education in collaboration with the American Medical Record Association. The majority of approved programs are at the undergraduate level and lead to a baccalaureate degree in medical record administration. A few approved programs exist whereby individuals who already have a baccalaureate degree may earn a certificate in medical record administration after twelve months of study. Successful completion of an approved program and the national examination enables the individual to bear the professional title of registered record administrator (R.R.A.).

MEDICAL RECORD ADMINISTRATION COURSE REQUIREMENTS

Course work in medical record administration consists of basic educational requirements in the humanities and the behavioral, biological, and physical sciences. Professional course work is a combination of theory and practical experience. The American Medical Association Council on Medical Education in collaboration with the American Medical Record Association has suggested that the curriculum include the following.*

Sciences
Anatomy and physiology
Medical terminology
Study of diseases in man

Medical record science
Medical record content, origin of clinical information
Identifying, numbering, filing, preserving, retrieving medical records
Standards for documentation
Classification systems, coding and indexing of diseases
Medical staff organization and functions
Techniques for evaluating clinical information

Management
Utilization and control of financial resources and budgets
Selection, utilization and control of space, supplies, equipment
Personnel administration
Wage and salary administration
Labor relations/unions
Inservice training
Professional communication skills

Information systems
Systems design and analysis
Development of information and management systems
Data processing
Record linkage
Application of computer concepts to the health field

*From American Medical Association Council on Medical Education in collaboration with American Medical Record Association: Proposed essentials of an accredited educational program for medical record administrators, Chicago, 1974, American Medical Association.

Legal aspects
Federal, state, and local laws and regulations
Security of health information
Moral and ethical control of health information
Confidentiality of health information

Health care delivery
Accreditation standards for a health care facility
Philosophy and objectives for governmental and community health care programs
Organizational patterns of a health care institution and agencies
Principles and practices of public health, local, state, and federal agencies
Current trends in health care delivery
Role and interrelationships of health care practitioners
Changing role of the health care provider

Research and statistical techniques

Clinical experience

Curriculums may vary from program to program.

QUALITIES OF A MEDICAL RECORD ADMINISTRATOR

Medical record administrators are professional managers responsible for a vital department in a health care facility. They must be able to lead the operation and motivate employees of a medical record department, guide other health professionals in the proper utilization and storage of patient information, communicate effectively both orally and in writing, be aggressive and willing to change as new technologies are discovered, and be organized in thought and performance. Accuracy and discretion are mandatory for the profession.

SUPPORTING PERSONNEL

Medical record administration is assisted by individuals trained in the technical skills of a medical record department. An accredited record technician (A.R.T.) performs departmental functions such as coding, indexing, and analyzing medical records and handling requests for the release of information. The A.R.T. may serve as a supervisor or assistant to the medical record administrator. In some facilities, the A.R.T. may act as a department head. Two types of educational programs exist for the A.R.T. One option is to enroll in an approved program for medical record technology in a two-year community or technical college. These two-year programs combine knowledge of medical record science with experiences in laboratory and health care facilities. The other educational option is the correspondence course offered by the American Medical Record Association. To participate in the correspondence course an individual must be working in a health care facility under the guidance of a registered record administrator. On successful completion of either one of these programs an individual is eligible to write the national examination for accredited record technician. On passing the examination, the individual is entitled to use the initials A.R.T.

JOB OPPORTUNITIES

Job opportunities for registered record administrators exist in all types of health care facilities. The R.R.A. may find employment outside the health care facility in commercial health insurance, computer, dictating equipment, data abstracting, and management consulting firms. Employment opportunities are available in government agencies from state health department divisions to the Veterans Administration. Registered record administrators are employed by the United States Public Health Service. Overseas employment may be obtained through organizations such as the Pan American World Health Organization. An R.R.A. may choose to be self-employed, consulting at nursing homes, small hospitals, doctors' offices, and other health care facilities that do not require a full-time R.R.A. Those interested in education may find teaching opportunities in educational institutions in both two- and four-year programs. The skills of the registered record administrator may be utilized by any organization dealing in patient information.

Compensation depends on the size, location, and type of employing facility or organization. Salaries tend to be higher in metropolitan areas. Average annual salaries range from $8,500 to $15,000; with experience, salaries may be as high as $25,000. The employment outlook for registered record administrators is excellent. As more emphasis is being placed on patient information and quality of care, more jobs are opening up for registered record administrators.

SUMMARY

Medical record administration is a challenging profession in which the medical record administrator plays an important role as member of the health care team. The need for properly documented medical information has flourished throughout the history of medicine. Recording of medical information has progressed from etchings on cave walls to written medical records. These medical records relate all that happens to a patient in a health care facility and serve to ensure that a patient receives quality health care. The responsibility of the medical record administrator is to oversee the recording, storing, retrieving, and handling of medical records in a patient information system. This responsibility includes the organization and management of a medical record department as well as patient information flow in a health care facility. Increasing demands to ensure quality patient care are placing more emphasis on the uses of medical records and the role of the medical record administrator. Medical record administration offers an individual a part in health care delivery and in a profession growing daily in terms of new technologies and excellent employment opportunities.

REFERENCES

American Medical Association Council on Medical Education in collaboration with American Medical Record Association: Proposed essentials of an accredited educational program for medical record administrators, Chicago, 1974, American Medical Association.

History of medical record science: from hieroglyphics to . . . electronic data processing, Medical Record News **40:**20, 1969.

Huffman, E. K.: Medical record management, ed. 6, Chicago, 1972, Physicians' Record Co.

Task force on the future role of the medical record administrator. Final report, April 9, 1974, Medical Record News **45:**66, 1974.

United States Department of Labor, Bureau of Labor Statistics: Employment outlook for medical record administrators, medical record technicians and clerks, Washington, D.C., 1974, United States Government Printing Office.

PROFESSIONAL ORGANIZATION WHERE FURTHER INFORMATION CAN BE OBTAINED

American Medical Record Association
875 North Michigan Avenue
Suite 1850, John Hancock Center
Chicago, Illinois, 60611

Chapter 11
Medical technology
Marjorie L. Brunner

Medical technology is one of the rapidly growing professions associated with modern advances in medical science. Medical technologists work in clinical pathology laboratories performing the scientific tests that track down the cause and cure of disease. Some diseases, diabetes and leukemia, for example, can be positively identified by laboratory methods alone, The presence of other suspected diseases can be confirmed by laboratory examination.

Medical technologists are prepared to function not only as laboratory workers but also as supervisors, instructors of supportive laboratory personnel, and researchers. They are educated and technically trained to perform the various chemical, microscopic, bacteriological, and other medical laboratory procedures used in the diagnosis, study, and treatment of disease. Medical technologists work under the supervision of a pathologist, a physician who specializes in laboratory medicine.

HOW DID MEDICAL TECHNOLOGY DEVELOP?

In the early days of clinical laboratory science, pathologists, who were just beginning to receive recognition as necessary and important medical specialists in their own right, performed their own laboratory tests. As the field of laboratory medicine developed and broadened, pathologists found it necessary to train assistants to help perform the simpler tests. The profession of medical technology thus came into being in the early part of this century.

In those years, high school graduates interested in medical technology commonly became apprentices in medical laboratories. Then a few commercial schools were established, but the training they offered was often inadequate, and their fees were usually exorbitant. Realizing that laboratory medicine was developing rapidly and that standards had to be established for the training of laboratory assistants, the American Society of Clinical Pathologists (ASCP) established the Board of Registry of Medical Technologists (ASCP) in 1928 and elected six pathologists to serve on the Board. The Registry administered the national certification examination to prospective medical technologists after they completed all educational requirements. The first certificates were issued in 1930.

The American Society for Medical Technology (ASMT) was organized in 1933. Membership was restricted to medical technologists certified by the Board of Registry. The present ASMT membership totals approximately 22,000. Today the Board of Registry of Medical Technologists (ASCP) consists of six members of ASCP and five members of ASMT.

In 1949 the ASCP formed a standing committee, the Board of Schools, to handle the accreditation of medical laboratory programs. The Board of Schools functioned until October, 1973, when the National Accrediting Agency for Clinical Laboratory Sciences (NAACLS) was created and co-sponsored by ASMT and ASCP. It assumed all the accreditation and transcript evaluation functions formerly held by the Board of Schools. NAACLS is composed of three medical technology educators active in ASMT, three clinical pathologist educators who are fellows of ASCP, two supportive-level practitioners, and six individuals elected by the above. By gradually elevating educational standards and improving the quality of technical training, both the Board of Registry and NAACLS have done much to raise the status of medical laboratory workers to a professional level.

WHERE DO MEDICAL TECHNOLOGISTS WORK? WHAT ARE THEIR CONTRIBUTIONS TO HEALTH CARE?

Clinical pathology laboratories, where most medical technologists are employed, include a variety of specialized areas. In the blood bank the medical technologist's knowledge and skill in matching blood samples are crucial. In addition to the familiar testing for blood groups and Rh factors, verifying that the patient's blood sample is compatible with the donor's blood can require from six to twenty highly sensitive and specific determinations.

In microbiology the greatest amount of work involves bacteria. The technologists grow and identify bacteria present in biological specimens obtained from patients and do tests to help determine which antibiotics will be most effective in subduing the organism causing the infection. (See Fig. 15.)

Problems in parasitology center on the search for an identification of parasites—the small animals living inside the body. These may be tapeworms or pinworms, or they may be tiny one-celled animals such as the parasite that causes malaria.

A knowledge of chemistry is used in many ways in medical laboratories. Technologists determine the presence and quantity of chemical substances in blood and other body fluids obtained from patients. Comparisons of the chemical constituents of patient specimens with normal values established in specimens from healthy individuals provide useful guides for the physician in his diagnosis and control of disease.

In serology the medical technologist uses standardized techniques to demonstrate the presence and amount of antibodies or antibody-like substances in body fluids such as serum, plasma, spinal fluid, and

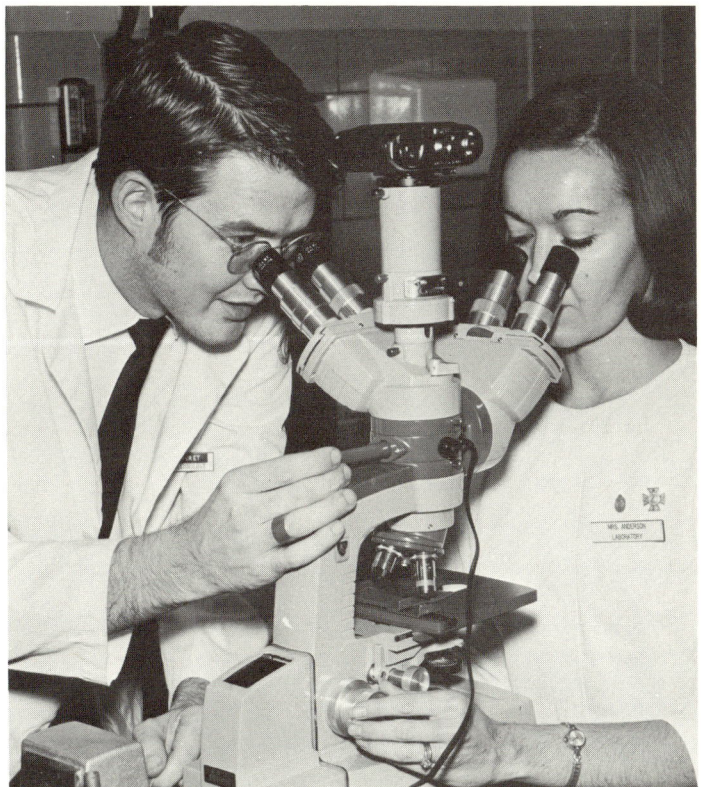

Fig. 15. Technologists in a microbiology laboratory examine a patient's specimen for the presence of bacteria.

urine. In many instances the production of these substances by the body has been stimulated by an infection or by immunization. The Widal test, for example, is used to demonstrate the presence of serum antibodies to *Salmonella typhosa*, which is the causative agent of typhoid fever.

Analyses of urine samples are beneficial in diagnosing or controlling illnesses caused by malfunction of the kidneys. Examination of urine specimens gives clues to such diseases as nephritis and diabetes. A potential new application for these tests is emerging through research into the biochemical conditions that are related to mental disorders.

In hematology, tests are conducted to detect conditions that primarily affect the blood, such as anemia (a deficiency of red blood cells commonly known as tired blood), hemophilia (a disease in which the blood clotting mechanism is defective), and leukemia (a type of cancer

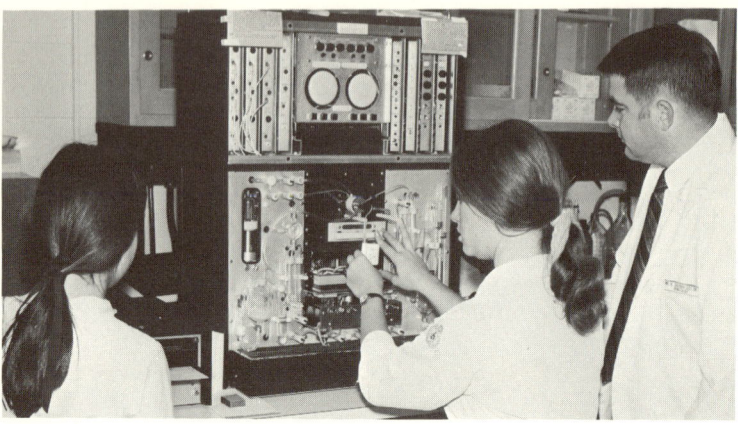

Fig. 16. Precision instruments are used to increase the accuracy and speed of blood counts performed in the hematology laboratory.

involving an abnormal increase in the number of white blood cells). (See Fig. 16.)

Work in a medical laboratory requires the use of a wide array of intricate precision equipment—microscopes, automatic analyzers that permit an increased number of patient fluid samples to be chemically analyzed with greater speed and accuracy, and electronic counters used for the enumeration of red and white blood cells. Specialized procedures such as electrophoresis and gas chromatography are used to isolate compounds present in body fluids so they may be identified and quantitated. New instruments and methods of analysis are constantly being developed, so that medical technologists are involved in an atmosphere of continuous learning, evaluation, and progress.

The types of positions available to the medical technologist are as varied as the many tests they perform. Laboratory work is being done in hospitals, clinics, doctors' offices, public health departments, and private research institutes as well as in industry. Those who prefer to watch the results of their work as it affects the health of specific individuals would probably prefer a position in a small hospital, clinic, or doctor's office, where they have an opportunity to get acquainted with the people they help. Other technologists may choose to work in research or industry, where their contributions may one day have a far-reaching effect on the health of many people.

Research positions that involve primarily routine laboratory techniques are often filled by supporting laboratory personnel such as certified laboratory assistants. However, research positions involving the development of new laboratory methods, the adaptation of existing methods to new equipment, and the evaluation of technical problems are available to experienced technologists in many clinical laboratories. Occasionally experienced technologists or those with advanced education work in basic research, an area that requires a good deal of initiative and independent thinking. They work closely with consultant pathologists or specialists in a related scientific field.

The following case study illustrates the contribution a medical technologist might make to the study, diagnosis, and treatment of a patient.

A 30-year-old expectant mother was seen by an obstetrician for prenatal care. Her medical history revealed that this was her fourth pregnancy. Her blood type was recorded as A, Rh negative, and her husband's blood type was O, Rh positive. Her first pregnancy had occurred when she was 23 years of age, and her baby was delivered after a full term of 40 weeks' gestation. The baby's blood type was O, Rh positive, and he was unaffected by the incompatibility of his parents' Rh factors. During the patient's second pregnancy, when she was 25 years of age, Rh antibodies present in her blood passed through the placenta into the baby's circulatory system, where they reacted with and destroyed some of the baby's red blood cells. The infant was delivered after 40 week's gestation and was given a blood transfusion to replenish his red blood cells. He responded well to this treatment. The patient's third pregnancy occurred at the age of 26 years. An Rh incompatibility was again apparent. The baby was given a blood transfusion after delivery at 40 weeks' gestation, but he failed to respond to this treatment and died soon after birth.

With this background information the obstetrician began to study his patient's condition. He requested that a medical technologist obtain blood samples from the patient and her husband to confirm their blood types. The medical technologist in the blood bank determined the patient's type as A, Rh negative, and the husband's type as O, Rh positive. The technologist also detected the presence of antibodies against the Rh factor in the patient's blood and determined further that the anitbody level was significant.

At 24 weeks' gestation the obstetrician collected a specimen of the amniotic fluid in which the baby was floating. This specimen was sent to the clinical laboratory, where another medical technologist performed a test that indicated the amount of red blood cell destruction present in the baby. This test was repeated at 26 weeks of gestation and again at 27 weeks because it seemed that the baby's condition was deteriorating. During the twenty-eighth week of gestation the obstetrician and pathologist decided that laboratory results of the amniotic fluid tests indicated the need for an intrauterine transfusion. Compatible blood was found and cross-matched by the medical technologist. The baby received a total of three transfusions in utero at 28, 30, and 32 weeks' gestation. Amniotic fluid was collected just prior to each transfusion. Part of this fluid was sent to the clinical bacteriology laboratory, where the medical technologist inoculated it onto media that would enhance the growth of any microorganisms present. Fortunately there were no indications of intrauterine infection.

At 36 weeks' gestation, labor was induced, and when the baby was delivered, blood samples were immediately collected from his umbilical cord and sent to the clinical laboratory. The medical technologist in the hematology laboratory performed blood cell counts and hemoglobin measurements to determine the degree of anemia present, and the medical technologist in the clinical chemistry laboratory made repeated measurements of the amount of bilirubin present in the blood. This is a compound produced by red blood cell destruction, and it can cause brain damage in the newborn infant if it is present in the blood in large quantities. Fortunately the level of bilirubin in this child's blood was only moderately elevated, and further blood transfusions were not necessary due to the protection the child had received through the intrauterine transfusions.

WHAT ARE THE EDUCATIONAL REQUIREMENTS?

Educational requirements for medical technology include a minimum of three years of college plus twelve months of clinical training in one of the 723 hospital laboratory schools of medical technology accredited by the Council on Medical Education of the AMA. Since January 1, 1962, the pretechnical educational requirements for admission to an approved school of medical technology have been three years (90 semester hours or 135 quarter hours) of course work in any accredited college or university. The student's program must include the following credits.

1. A minimum of sixteen semester hours (twenty-four quarter hours) of chemistry are required. Organic chemistry or biological chemistry must be included. Quantitative analysis and physical chemistry are recommended.
2. A minimum of sixteen semester hours (twenty-four quarter hours) of biological science are required. Microbiology must be included. Immunology, genetics, physiology, and anatomy are recommended.
3. A minimum of one semester or quarter of college-level mathematics is required. Courses in statistics and physics are strongly recommended.

The college or university should accept this course work toward the first three years of a baccalaureate program in medical technology. Some of the approved schools of medical technology have their own specific course requirements in addition to those mentioned.

After earning the necessary college credits, students must satisfactorily complete a course of instruction in all phases of medical technology at an approved school. Major topics of instruction include hematology, urinalysis, clinical microbiology, serology, immunology, blood banking, and clinical chemistry. After completing these professional education requirements, students must be eligible for a baccalaureate degree. In order to become registered medical technologists-- M.T.(ASCP)—students must pass the examination administered by the Board of Registry of Medical Technologists (ASCP).

There are also advanced educational programs for medical technologists who wish to obtain categorical certification in one particular field. For example, the certification program of the American Association of Blood Banks is designed to train specialists in blood banking. This program is offered only by institutions that have been approved by the association and consists of one year of training. This program includes both didactic study and practical experience and is designed to provide a comprehensive education in all aspects of the modern-day blood bank. After completing the course, all candidates for certification must take the examination that is given once each year by the Board of Registry of Medical Technologists (ASCP) in cooperation with the Committee on Education of the American Association of Blood Banks. The examination consists of written and practical portions, and both must be passed in the same year. The technologist then becomes a certified blood bank specialist—M.T.(ASCP)B.B. There are also certification programs in chemistry, microbiology, and hematology. Since these specialists are expected to have a wide range of competence and a thorough understanding of their particular fields, they often become supervisors or work in advanced research projects or special reference laboratories.

Students planning a career in medical technology should consider the possibility of pursuing a graduate degree. Graduate education is assuming increasing importance as necessary preparation for the more interesting job opportunities. Specialist certification in hematology, microbiology, or chemistry is available by examination for those with a master's or doctoral degree in the specialty and/or the required years of experience. Information concerning graduate programs in medical technology is available through the NAACLS.

WHAT PARTICULAR QUALITIES ARE NEEDED?

A list of qualifications for a career in medical technology might include an interest in and aptitude for science, an active curiosity, the ability to work under pressure, manual dexterity, and a general desire to help mankind. Self-discipline, a spirit of cooperation, and thorough moral and intellectual integrity are essential in the practice of this profession. The laboratory findings obtained by medical technologists are used in making vital decisions concerning human lives. Therefore procedures must be performed with accuracy and the result evaluated with the utmost integrity.

WHO ARE THE SUPPORTING PROFESSIONALS IN MEDICAL LABORATORIES?

There are many workers in medical laboratories whose educational backgrounds are more limited than those of medical technologists. Nonetheless, they are trained to perform necessary and valuable services in the laboratory. Certified laboratory assistants are capable of handling a variety of procedures under the supervision of a medical technologist. Their tasks may range from collecting blood specimens to operating modern and complex equipment. Educational requirements for certified laboratory assistants include a diploma from an accredited high school plus twelve months of training in one of the 182 AMA-approved hospital schools for certified laboratory assistants. Training includes lectures and applied laboratory training, and students who complete the program are eligible to take the national examination given by the Board of Registry of Medical Technologists (ASCP). Those who pass the examination become certified laboratory assistants—C.L.A.(ASCP). Proficiency examinations for clinical laboratory personnel or basic military medical laboratory courses and appropriate experience may replace the training programs just described.

A second supporting professional in a medical laboratory is the cytotechnologist. Cytotechnologists are concerned with cytology, the science of cells, and are trained to recognize those minute abnormalities in the size, shape, and color of cell substances that may signal the presence of cancer. Their main tool is the microscope, and a variety of special stains are used to accentuate cell patterns. Cytotechnologists must complete two years of college, including twelve semester hours in biology, plus twelve months of training at one of nearly 100 schools of cytotechnology approved by the AMA. After candidates pass the examination given by the Board of Registry of Medical Technologists (ASCP), they become cytotechnologists—C.T.(ASCP).

Histologic technicians are also members of the medical laboratory team. They prepare portions of selected body tissues for microscopic examination. Tissue preparation involves freezing and cutting tissue samples into ultrathin slices, mounting them on slides, and staining them with special dyes to make cell details more clearly visible under the microscope. Histologic technicians must have a high school diploma plus one year of supervised training in a qualified pathology laboratory or graduation from one of the twenty-six programs of histologic technique approved by the AMA. After certification through examination by the Board of Registry of Medical Technologists, histologic technicians are given the designation H.T.(ASCP).

Medical laboratory technicians are the most recently established category of supporting professionals in a medical laboratory. The level of responsibility that can be assumed by the medical laboratory technician lies between that of the certified laboratory assistant and the medical technologist. Two-year programs leading to an associate degree for medical laboratory technicians are presently being established. Nineteen such programs have been approved by the AMA. Certification as medical laboratory technicians—M.L.T.(ASCP)—is available to those who successfully complete the certification examination given by the Board of Registry (ASCP).

Nuclear medical technologists assist the physician in the operation of scanning devices using radioisotopes. The educational and experience requirements for acceptance to take the Registry examination are varied and may be obtained from the Board of Registry of Medical Technologists (ASCP).

WHAT CAN LABORATORY PERSONNEL EXPECT TO EARN?

Starting salaries earned by laboratory personnel vary according to the level of their training and performance and are also determined in part by the size of the employing facility and its geographical location. The federal government paid newly graduated medical technologists with bachelor's degrees annual starting salaries of $7,694 in early 1973. Those having experience, superior academic achievement, or one year of graduate study began at $9,520. The ASMT 1974 National Salary Survey determined that the mean yearly salary for a staff technologist was $8,292. The same study showed a mean annual salary for cytotechnologists of $7,692. Medical laboratory technicians averaged $6,072, histologic technicians averaged $5,460, and laboratory assistants averaged $4,872 annually.

WHAT IS THE DEMAND FOR MEDICAL TECHNOLOGISTS?

A career in medical technology is both stimulating and rewarding. Although a majority of the approximately 60,000 ASCP-registered medical technologists are women, the number of men entering the profession is increasing rapidly. The growing dependence on laboratory tests in the diagnosis and treatment of disease as well as the construction of more hospital and medical facilities have increased the demand for medical technologists. It is estimated that 90,000 professional medical technologists will be needed by 1978. Registered medical technologists will find opportunities for employment in every part of the country.

REFERENCES

Allied Medical Education Directory, Chicago, 1974, American Medical Association.

The Registry of Medical Technologists of the American Society of Clinical Pathologists, Chicago, 1969, Board of Registry of medical Technologists, American Society of Clinical Pathologists.

What kind of a career could I have in a medical laboratory? Chicago, no date, Board of Registry of Medical Technologists, American Society of Clinical Pathologists.

SUGGESTED READING

Williams, M. R.: Introduction to medical technology, Philadelphia, 1971, Lea & Febiger.

PROFESSIONAL ORGANIZATIONS WHERE FURTHER INFORMATION CAN BE OBTAINED

American Society of Clinical Pathologists
2100 W. Harrison Street
Chicago, Illinois 60612

Registry of Medical Technologists of ASCP
Box 4872
Chicago, Illinois 60680

**American Society for Medical
 Technology**
Suite 200
5555 West Loop South
Bellaire, Texas 77401

**National Accrediting Agency for
 Clinical Laboratory Sciences**
Suite 1512
222 South Riverside Plaza
Chicago, Illinois 60606

Chapter 12
Medicine
George L. Fite

THE VARIETIES OF MEDICAL PRACTICE

The profession of medicine as we know it today has developed from early practices rooted in magic and superstition, herbalism, bloodletting, and folk medicine. Nurtured by the knowledge of the early European universities, supported by practices rooted in cultural biases, and divided by differing beliefs regarding the basic functions of the human organism, the profession of medicine has managed to evolve as both a healing art and an essential science.

Remnants of the early differences of opinion still survive, resulting in sectarianism in medicine, specifically homeopathic, osteopathic, and allopathic. No realist can expect these forces to be wholly extinguished, but their histories have shown a steady departure from their origins into union with the majority to form an eclectic discipline.

Homeopathy as taught by the German-born Samuel Hahnemann at one time enjoyed a large following. According to this discipline, all diseases were to be treated by the administration of minute doses of drugs that would produce the symptoms of the particular disease if the particular drug were given to a healthy person. Hahnemann Medical College and Hospital was founded in 1848 and still flourishes in Philadelphia. Although token recognition is given to the homeopathic philosophy, the school now is a standard medical educational institution.

Osteopathic medicine tends to merge similarly with standard academic medicine but has resisted attempts at organizational merger and remains a practice differentiated by its underlying emphasis on the importance of the musculoskeletal system in the body's efforts to resist and overcome disease. Its basic scientific knowledge and its system of medical education have indeed moved toward the standard practice in diagnostic, preventive, and therapeutic procedures, but its practitioners always maintain their focus on the musculoskeletal system and its effect on neurophysiologic processes. Osteopathic physicians maintain a separate organizational identity and tend to be involved in general practice more than in the specialties.

Allopathic medicine, the third and most widespread branch of modern medicine, is based on the premise that a disease process can be altered by action against the causative agent. An example would be the reduction of bacterial infection through the action of penicillin.

The practice of modern medicine not only derives from these different approaches but also is affected by new interests such as that presently appearing in North America in the practice of acupuncture, which to some holds great promise. This ancient technology, new to our culture, has become interwoven with modern technology and exemplifies the way in which the outer reaches of medical practice invite scientific investigation to produce imaginative proposals for the prevention or cure of all disease.

Primary physicians

Home-visiting doctors have disappeared from our cities and most of our country, as have their turn-of-the-century buckboards and little black bags. Neither hitching post nor automobile parking space is available for them today. The problem of primary care is better described as a problem in logistic medicine, the delivery of health care to the patient. It is medicine's business to support health in the community before signs and symptoms appear; hence the primary physician (rather than the general practitioner) who can guide the patient to advanced inquiry and treatment, if the physician cannot provide it himself. Primary physicians are badly needed in many sparsely settled and low-income communities. Their incomes may be smaller than those of their specialist colleagues, and their work may be hard and their hours long. Of today's medical school graduates hardly a third look in this direction.

Family physicians

Closely related to the primary physician is the family physician. The distinction may be superficial, yet internships are today offered in family medicine, and the existence of an academy of family medicine, recognizing the field as a specialty, suggests that the primary physician is beginning to find leadership next door. In both of these fields, where patients are in need of much examination that does not demand the physician's skills, the *physician's assistant* emerges as a force in the delivery of health care. (The profession of physician's assistant is discussed in Chapter 18.)

Specialties

The road to a specialty begins in medical school, and the sooner students choose their specialty, the smoother their progress. Only a minority makes this decision quickly or early. In the last academic years and in internships, electives help specialty-bound physicians to find their field. The specialties* are themselves highly organized, and they require examination before their boards prior to admission. Although some have charged specialty groups with similarity to the guilds

---

*Specialties are listed in Appendix B.

of western Europe during the Middle Ages, the standards they set are high. Few hospitals, clinics, or group practices will accept specialists who either have not passed board examinations in their specialty or are eligible to become so certified.

Group practice

The gathering together of specialists into a unit capable of handling most medical problems has developed naturally from its predecessor, the hospital outpatient department. The advantages of group practice to both patient and doctor usually include the all-important availability of hospital beds when needed. Indeed, some hospitals have originated and developed from the needs prescribed by group practices.

As small businessmen, many doctors finds themselves involved in things for which they have no real taste. These include the purchase of expensive equipment, office rentals, finding secretarial-receptionist help and nursing aides, and problems with taxation, insurance, and fee collection. The larger private clinic or group practice can enjoy an administrative staff, freeing the physician from nonmedical duties. Partnership in group practice usually includes retirement provisions and vacation coverage. Possible disadvantages are that the group practitioner will lose some of his individuality and freedom for personalized behavior.

Military and government service

The armed forces and the United States Public Health Service offer career positions to physicians as commissioned officers. Several thousands of doctors find this service helpful in repaying the heavy debts acquired during their educations. The extensive hospital system of the Veterans Administration is a large employer of physicians. These large institutions relieve physicians of their role as family counselor, giving them more time to follow personal medical interests. State and county health societies employ many physicians, not always on a full-time basis, as do insurance companies.

Foundation medicine

The largest research organization in the world is the National Institutes of Health (NIH) in Bethesda, Maryland. It is federally owned and operated by the Department of Health, Education, and Welfare. The NIH is a massive laboratory of investigative medicine and employs hundreds of chemists, physicists, and scientists knowledgeable in all fields of biology and medicine. Other examples of research institutions are the Communicable Diseases Center in Atlanta, the Rockefeller University (formerly the Rockefeller Institute of Medical Research) in New York City, and the American Cancer Society, which channels funds from both public and private sources into the support of advances in research, patient care, and treatment throughout the country. Scores of

other foundations attack many individual diseases, and commercial firms also support private research along the lines of their own interests.

HUMAN VALUES IN MEDICINE

Hippocrates, often called the father of medicine, enjoyed a flourishing general practice on the island of Cos following his study in Athens. This was 400 years before the birth of Christ and 2,000 years prior to the beginnings of a correct understanding of physiology. The Hippocratic oath, probably written some years after his death, reflects the importance of impeccable behavior on the part of the physician toward medical colleagues as well as patients. Somewhat pious in tone, its

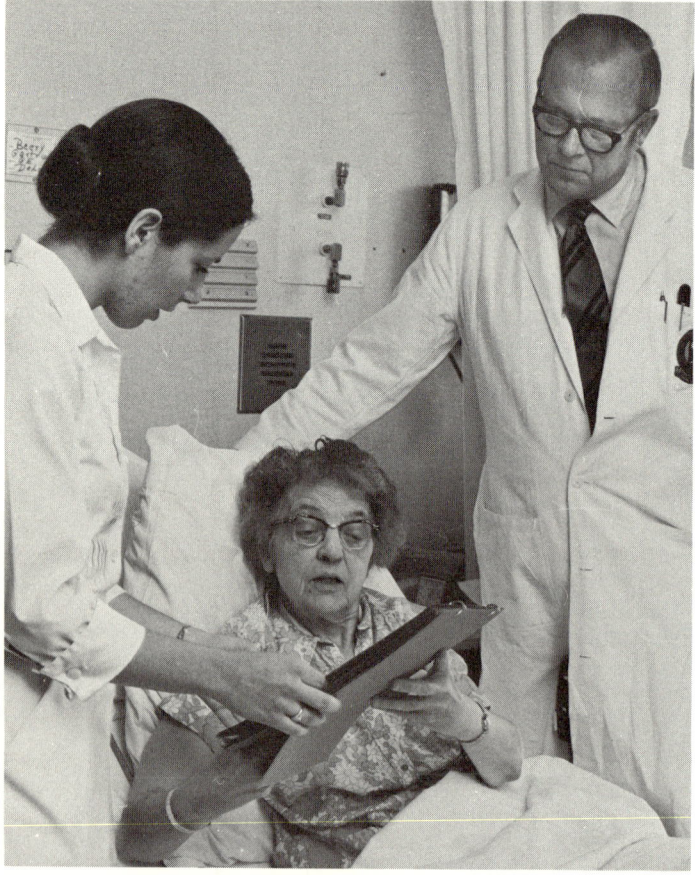

Fig. 17. Physicians develop treatment plans in conference with other members of the health care team, in this case a dietitian and the patient.

concept of the "good physician" remains essentially unchanged today, so much so that the oath is commonly recited at medical school graduation exercises as a declaration of moral fiber and as a recognition of the human responsibilities of the physician. Revisions have been suggested to adapt the oath to the modern scene, while articles about the "good physician" still appear in medical journals, and relicensure of doctors and continuing medical education are demanded.

The ethical dilemma of modern medicine is that the endeavor to save one life often involves human judgments concerning other lives and other values. This conflict is seen in the kidney transplant candidate waiting for a suitable cadaver kidney, in the woman seeking an abortion, in the mechanical prolongation of life where meaning and humanness have ceased.

Medical knowledge acquired during the past twenty years exceeds *in quantity* all that acquired earlier. What sort of resolutions will the physicians of today and tomorrow find for the dilemmas that have already begun to occur at the interface of technology and human values? (See Fig. 17.)

MEDICAL EDUCATION

America's first medical school opened its doors 200 years ago. Medical education in the United States developed slowly during its first 100 years and was greatly influenced by European medicine throughout the nineteeth century. Only after World War I did medical education in the United States come to occupy a position of leadership.

Teaching programs in United States medical schools vary only slightly from school to school. The fifty-year standard has been the study of basic sciences during the first two years, with clinical medicine and bedside experience the focus of the second two years. This division has permitted the existence of the two-year school, which offered only the subjects standard to the first half of the process, sometimes because resources were not great enough to meet the demands of clinical education.

The basic sciences commonly taught in the first year of medical school are gross and microscopic anatomy, human physiology, biological chemistry, and pharmacology. During the second year students are introduced to the disease process. They will experience prolonged classroom and laboratory instruction in microbiology, including bacteriology, virology, the study of fungi, parasites, and all related agencies of infectious disease. In addition, in pathology they will be taught both the gross and microscopic anatomy of disease processes and will learn their epidemiological and genetic backgrounds and applications in sanitation, public health, and practical immunology.

During these two years their interest in medicine and its practice will be steadily stimulated by some introduction to and exhibition of the clinical process, but they will have little direct involvement in this aspect. They will be hard put to absorb and retain what they have been taught.

After these two years students are eligible to take Part I of the National Board Examinations and will probably do so at this time when their knowledge of the subject is freshest.

Teaching the basic sciences has been a subject for considerable academic debate. Obviously, the student who is to become a psychiatrist or ophthalmologist will have spent many hours learning things that will seem forever useless. Potential cardiologists may easily lament time given to the study of tropical diseases, cases of which they will never see. Fifteen years ago, therefore, some schools relaxed their teachings of basic sciences, introducing clinical medicine as a replacement. The results were not altogether happy; too many students even from the best medical schools were unable to pass their National Board examinations. The tide has recently reversed, and the basic sciences have been reinstated. To say that the problem has been resolved is false. Behind the problem lies the enormous fund of information to be assimilated as well as the difficulty of presenting the material in ways appropriate to individual needs.

Within the past five years, nearly a third of the medical schools have introduced accelerated curriculums. In general, these changes have redesigned the basic and introductory clinical sciences of the traditional first two years so as to follow body systems in presentation. To reduce the amount of time spent in academic preparation, vacations have virtually been eliminated for students who complete the total M.D. requirements in three years. Many programs have added some flexibility in time and a few have introduced innovative independent study programs that allow for considerable variation in self-pacing through the basic sciences.

During their third year medical students spend much time in the outpatient clinic, within many or all of its divisions. Under supervision they will examine many patients, working together with a few colleagues in comparatively small groups. They will still be students, even though their white coats, stethoscopes, and pocketfuls of throat sticks give them the appearance of doctors.

Students will be introduced to most of the specialties, perhaps all of them. In addition, they will be intensely lectured to, both didactically and with amphitheater demonstration, and will have difficulty in keeping up with as much as they could wish. They will begin to discover the fields that interest them most, surely giving more time to these at the expense of others.

In their fourth year students will enter the hospital wards, spending much time in many of the byways of the hospital, its laboratories, its meetings, its ward rounds, its surgeries, its radiologic areas. They will take the ward patient histories, be mercilessly scouted by the residents, and be put through what may well turn out to have been the most fascinating year of their lives.

Then they will receive the degree of doctor of medicine and be permitted to take the second part of the National Board examinations. But they cannot yet practice medicine. Some states require service of one or two years in hospital internship or residency as a requisite to licensure. Thus, armed with their degrees, physicians are still many months away from independent practice.

Licensure to practice medicine is required by all states, and all demand examination of the candidate. All but two states have now joined the FLEX group and use an identical examination given at the same time each year. Questions for this examination are chosen from the National Board pool, and the grading is weighted so that basic sciences count one sixth, clinical sciences count one third, and clinical problem-solving questions count one half in final grade computation. Reciprocity, better termed *licensure by endorsement,* is facilitated and made more uniform by this cooperative testing mechanism. However, it should be noted that each state maintains its own individual passing score for licensure.

PREREQUISITES FOR MEDICAL SCHOOL ADMISSION

Fifty years ago many educators thought the entering medical student should have a broad background in literature, language, and the fine arts. They wanted the students with a proven aptitude and capacity for learning—"We'll teach them the rest."

Medical schools still want the student with aptitude and zeal, but the prerequisites for the basic science portion of the curriculum are too many and too essential for the school to accept a candidate without them.

Prospective physicians must start to acquire the prerequisites two to three years before applying to medical school. Whether or not they eventually enter medicine, their decision to prepare cannot wait, and their eligibility for entry to medical school will drop progressively if they procrastinate. Today's medical school asks that the entering student be prepared for the maximum course load, and it has come as a substantial shock to many beginners to discover that what they considered a heavy load in college was only recreation. If medical school candidates were not sufficiently motivated to have started early, their handicap becomes evident. Potential dropouts are costly risks to the school, and they are mercilessly screened out, especially because the demand for entry far exceeds available places.

Premedical preparatory courses cannot be specifically listed. Because microbiology is emphasized in medical school, a limited course in college bacteriology would not be important. A reading knowledge of French and German means less today than a grasp of calculus, and without a solid background in physics, organic chemistry, and genetic biology medical students are behind in their capacity to absorb what is offered them and to produce what is demanded.

There is no trend back to "The Doctor" as portrayed by Sir Luke Fildes, copied in a 1947 United States postage stamp, in which the doctor sits with chin on hand studying a sick child. An irreverent medical student has commented, "He can't figure the kid out, and is waiting for the rescue squad to take over." The compassionately correct approach is not enough. The demands of the practice of medicine also apply to premedical preparation.

FOREIGN MEDICAL SCHOOLS

Of the several thousand annual disappointed applicants to medical schools in the United States, many hundreds seek admission to foreign medical schools, especially those in France and Mexico. Although their qualifications may not be as high as those of the accepted applicants, many of the better applicants are as eligible as some of those accepted and are wholly competent to become doctors. Among the better, success is the rule. The road is rough, expensive, and long.

At one time tuition fees in foreign schools were low, but they have risen. In Mexico, United States students pay fees much higher than those assessed their Mexican classmates, and the total costs will be comparable to those of the average school at home, perhaps higher. The language problem has not been an obstacle, except as regards the time required to learn the foreign tongue.

The major stumbling block has been that foreign medical schools do not provide clinical training demanded of United States returnees after graduation from a foreign medical school. Before being permitted to practice in the United States, graduates of foreign medical schools must pass an examination given by the Educational Council for Foreign Medical Graduates (ECFMG). They must have a foreign license. To obtain a license in Mexico, graduates must give a year to a Mexican internship and another to Mexico's social service. They may succeed in bypassing some of this, but foreign medical graduates have not always been welcome as interns in United States teaching hospitals because of lack of experience in direct patient care. Alternate pathways, serving as an assistant to a practicing physician, for example, have not yet become real possibilities.

Still it is something of a tribute to the determination and the character of these students that a great many do catch up with their United States–educated colleagues, achieving full equality. The cost is high in money and in time.

Foreign medical schools, aware of all this and wishing to promote the best in medicine, have raised admissions standards, thereby reducing the percentage of dropouts. They seek to expand teaching in clinical medicine, although facilities are painfully inadequate. The ECFMG examinations emphasize knowledge in clinical medicine.

Meanwhile, the rising number of United States medical schools and their increasing numbers of students will increase the supply of doctors, supplemented as at the moment by numerous native graduates from many foreign countries. In the end, United States medical schools should supply adequate numbers of doctors, for the present number of qualified applicants to medical schools is large enough to provide the doctors needed. The certification of United States graduates of foreign medical schools will at that point be a problem only in individuals, rather than to the many now affected.

MEDICAL MISTAKES AND THE DOCTOR'S DILEMMA

Today's physician-surgeons are beset with legal problems. They are legally obligated to practice the skills normal to the procedure they perform, whether surgical, pharmacological, or other. They may make an honest mistake without penalty, provided that they have used all the medical skill inherent and common to the art or the surgery they have practiced. Determination of what may reasonably be expected of them is arguable, and determination of penalty in case of fault is a decision made by a jury subjected to emotional as well as medical demands. "Malpractice" is a current multimillion dollar football game, with lawyers the offensive coaches and doctors the defensive players.

Protective insurance, once available at an annual cost of $4,500 to the practitioner, has doubled or tripled. A recent news item told of the retirement of an active orthopedist when he was required to pay a $14,000 annual fee for malpractice insurance. A major company refuses to insure except against claims filed within the insurance year, but many claims arise many months or years after the fact. Still another major insurer against malpractice has retired from the field altogether.

The future of this moderately insane situation will be substantially affected by the increasing involvement of the federal government in medicine. Will a national health insurance act additionally insure the the physician against malpractice judgments? An honest physician doing his best can today be made bankrupt by a judgment in the hundreds of thousands of dollars, more than he might earn in a lifetime. Not even the best in competence and utmost in caution can rid the doctor of this dilemma. Current physician self-improvement regulations (PSROs) enacted by the government have not eased the problem and thus far offer little promise.

Big malpractice awards have grown enormously, as have suits. Fifteen thousand suits are expected in 1975 and following years. The newly graduated physician can expect to be sued once or twice in his career. Hospitals do not escape, nor do manufacurers of devices that have failed or caused injury. In the end the malpractice judgment is charged back to the patient in higher fees, but not to the same patient. Group practices and medical societies succeed in averaging things out, but the incongruous problem persists.

WOMEN PHYSICIANS

The steady increase in the number of women physicians and in the number of women entering medical schools suggests that in the 1990s at least a fifth of the physicians practicing in the United States will be women. Approximately one fourth of the new admissions to the Harvard Medical School are now women, and the increase is spreading broadly. The ratio is still far below that in the Soviet Union, where every other physician is a woman.

Prejudices against "lady doctors" and "henmedics" have changed, but the lion that wears the mane still likes to roar. His voice, now a growl, has not yielded to equal rights movements or feminism but to the obvious realization that a woman who can be a capable mother, secretary, nurse, or administrator, qualifies similarly as a physician. Prejudice against women arises occasionally in the argument that women can not effectively examine and treat male patients for venereal disease, however effective they may be as pediatricians. These same prejudices have not been voiced regarding male obstetricians and gynecologists.

In practice, the woman physician's difficulties in patient relationships dissolve quickly in the light of competence and understanding. In the end, the effectiveness of the prescription counts, not the handwriting thereof.

SUMMARY

The prospective medical student has many fields of practice from which to choose. The years of study and clinical training require careful preparation and single-minded concentration, demanding at the same time an awareness of human values and the development of the young physician's own values together with clinical skills.

SUGGESTED READINGS

Howe, H. F., editor: The physician's career, Chicago, 1967, American Medical Association.

Knight, J. A.: Medical student, doctor in the making, New York, 1973, Meredith Corp.

Lipkin, M: The care of patients, concepts and tactics, New York, 1974, Oxford University Press, Inc.

Journal of the American Osteopathic Association, Education Annual **72** (suppl.): entire issue, 1973.

PROFESSIONAL ORGANIZATIONS WHERE FURTHER INFORMATION CAN BE OBTAINED

American Medical Association
535 North Dearborn Street
Chicago, Illinois 60610

American Osteopathic Association
212 East Ohio Street
Chicago, Illinois 60611

Chapter 13
Nursing and related programs

Nursing
Katherine L. Kisker

HISTORICAL PERSPECTIVE

The real beginnings of nursing, contrary to popular belief, can be traced far beyond the mid-nineteenth century, for nursing is a profession that is almost as old as civilization. There are references to nursing in writings of the ancient Egyptians, Greeks, and Persians. In India, for example, there were training programs for nurses as early as 300 B.C. The word "nurse" is derived from the Latin word *nutrio*, which means to nourish and nurture, and these seem to have been the principal activities of nurses at that time.

Very little was done to improve the quality of nursing until the "Nightingale era" in the mid-1850s. In fact, in the early 1800s nurses in European countries often had an unfavorable reputation and seem to have been concerned mainly with their own personal gain. Few had any real education. Florence Nightingale was a well-educated woman, although she had received only a few weeks of formal training in nursing. Deeply concerned with social and health reforms in England, she endowed a training school for nurses in that country and was instrumental in planning the curriculum and selecting the students. The influence of her successful program spread throughout England and eventually to the United States, where in 1872 the first class of trained nurses was graduated from the New England Hospital for Women and Children in Boston. Nursing education began to move into the university setting in 1909, when the first collegiate school was established at the University of Minnesota.

Many social changes have occurred since the first nursing programs were developed in the United States, and these changes continue to have a great influence on both nursing practice and nursing education.

NURSES' CONTRIBUTIONS TO HEALTH CARE

Nursing practice involves several essential areas of patient care. Nurses are most frequently associated with physical care, for they provide or supervise the care that patients need because of illness or disability. This includes supplying what is necessary for the patient's safety and comfort as well as helping to prevent complications that may occur as a result of illness or measures used in treating it.

91

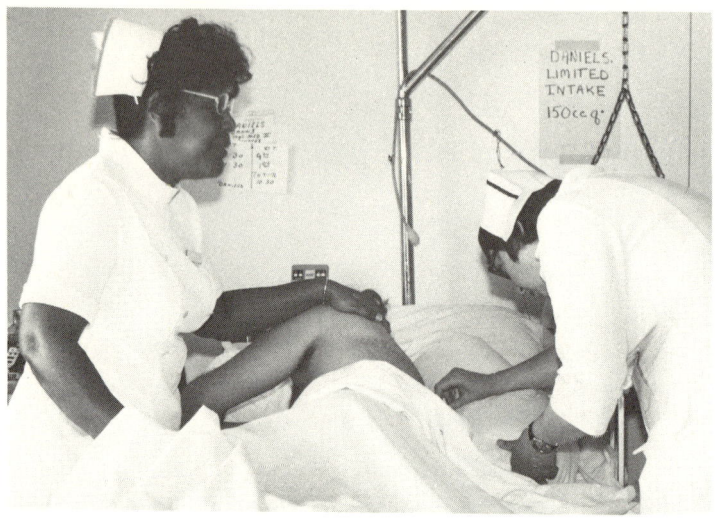

Fig. 18. Turning patients regularly and checking skin for pressure sores are essential parts of nursing care for patients who are unable to turn themselves.

A second function is that of providing emotional support. The nurse helps patients to understand and to express their feelings about their illness and what it may mean to their everyday existence. This understanding may strongly contribute to recovery and rehabilitation.

The education and experience of registered nurses enables them to make observations that are invaluable in patient care. They generally are the only health professionals who have contact with the patient on a twenty-four hour basis. The ability to recognize and note facts concerning the patient's condition, to act on the basis of these observations, and to communicate them to appropriate persons on the health team may be critical to the patient's recovery.

Nurses are also responsible for executing treatments that have been ordered by the physician. This requires a combination of technical skills and knowledge of the procedure, together with an understanding of its expected results. (See Fig. 18.)

Teaching patients and their families about an illness and the treatment measures used to combat it involves another important area of nursing. The instruction, whether planned or incidental, must be based on the knowledge and previous experience of those receiving it. The nurse is sensitive to the most appropriate time for giving such information as well as to the manner in which it is given.

Another function is that of conferring with other health team members, patients, and their families so that all patient services can be coordinated and so that all those involved work toward the same

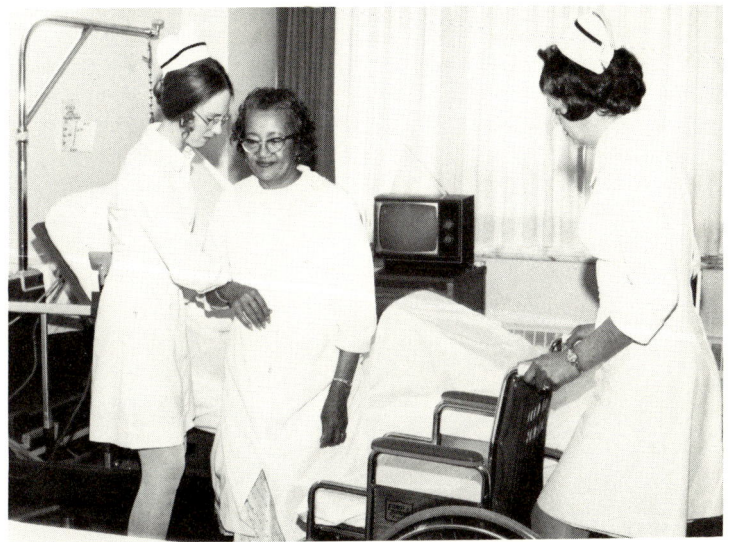

Fig. 19. Nurses help a surgical patient transfer from bed to chair.

ultimate goal. Because they observe and interact with the patient in an ongoing manner, nurses are good sources for the information that other members of the health team need in order to make their most effective contribution to the patient's care. (See Fig. 19.)

Other important responsibilities of nursing practice lie in the areas of health maintenance and disease prevention, which are receiving much more emphasis in the health care delivery system of today.

EDUCATIONAL REQUIREMENTS FOR THE REGISTERED NURSE

The three types of programs that prepare students to become registered nurses are the diploma program, the baccalaureate degree program, and the associate degree program. The oldest and most common are diploma programs, which are sponsored by and situated in hospitals. Diploma programs are generally three years in length. In some instances they are affiliated with colleges where the students take basic science and liberal arts courses, while in other instances all instruction is given at the hospital school. These programs emphasize instruction and related clinical experience that focus on the care of hospitalized patients. Part of the cost of a diploma school education may be borne by the sponsoring hospital itself. In recent years a number of diploma programs have been phased out and additional baccalaureate and associate degree programs have been developed in areas where diploma schools once were in operation.

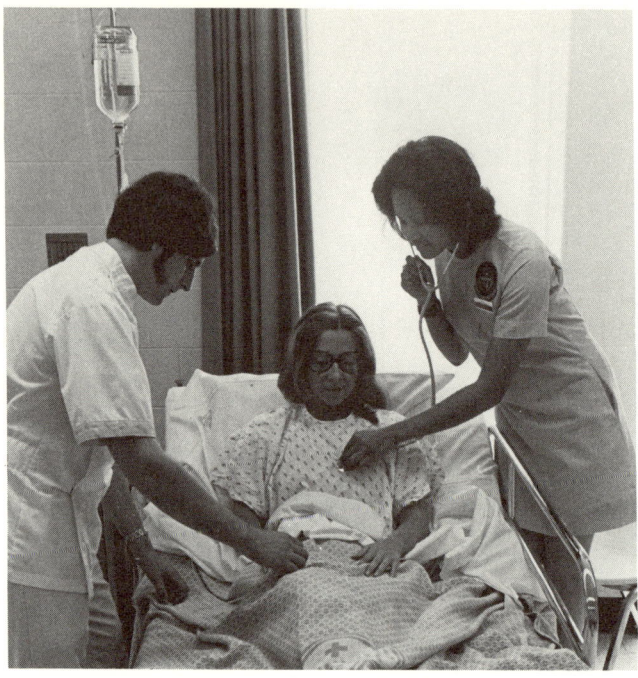

Fig. 20. Two student nurses check a newly admitted patient. (Courtesy The Ohio State University.)

The second type of program is the baccalaureate program, which offers a bachelor of science degree in nursing. Graduates of these programs are prepared as professional nurses and assume job responsibilities in a wide variety of health care delivery systems. Baccalaureate programs are designed to give the student a wide variety of educational experiences as well as the knowledge and skills specific to nursing. In most baccalaureate curriculums nursing courses and related supporting courses (for example, anatomy and physiology) account for somewhat more than half of the total credit hours required for graduation. The remaining credits needed for graduation are drawn from related biological, physical, and social sciences, the humanities, and electives. The programs vary in length from four to five academic years.

The third type of program is the associate degree program, which may be offered through a community college, technical institute, or university. The graduate of this program is prepared as a technical nurse and may find a more narrow range of job opportunities than the graduate of a baccalaureate program. Associate degree programs are generally two years in length and provide the student with basic courses in the physical, biological, and social sciences and the humanities. The nursing courses provide nursing theory and practice experiences.

The most likely trend for the future of nursing education is moving all nursing programs in the direction of degree-granting programs, that is, associate degree and baccalaureate programs. Many diploma schools have been phased out, and many new associate degree and baccalaureate programs have been developed. (See Fig. 20.)

Many nursing schools are looking critically at how different types of educational programs articulate to assist in the upward educational mobility of nurses. At the present time there are only a few programs that allow this process to occur at a high level.

Admission requirements to schools of nursing vary. Although many schools require college preparatory work at the high school level, it is advisable to contact specific schools to determine their requirements. The costs of programs vary depending on the nature of the institution of which they are a part.

The graduates of all three types of programs qualify to take a licensing examination. Graduates who pass these examinations are entitled to be licensed to practice as registered nurses. The requirements for licensure are determined by each state, and at the present time all states are using the same examination, although this practice may change in the future.

Preparation for positions in teaching, nursing administration, and clinical specialties is available at the master's degree level. Graduates of diploma and associate degree programs must earn a baccalaureate degree prior to pursuing a master's degree.

A listing of the programs accredited by the National League for Nursing (NLN) can be obtained by writing to the League at 10 Columbus Circle, New York, New York 10019. This listing is also published in the organization's journal, *Nursing Outlook.*

JOB OPPORTUNITIES

Graduates of all three types of programs have a variety of employment opportunities. The extent to which nurses are able to assess a patient's needs, carry out nursing care, and function with other health professionals is determined by their own abilities and motivation, educational background, experience, and the policies of the employing agency.

Nurses are employed in a wide variety of settings. General hospitals employ the greatest number of nurses; within their confines the nurse may work in the emergency room, operating room, intensive care units, delivery room, nursery, patient care units, or in many specialized areas where nursing care is needed. Nurses may also work in outpatient departments, extended care facilities, clinics, doctors' offices, psychiatric care settings, schools, industries, public health agencies, and numerous other settings where health and health care are areas of concern. If nurses choose to be self-employed, they may become private-duty nurses or independent nurse practitioners.

Three of these areas of nursing practice will be discussed in more detail to provide an idea of the nature of these fields and the skills needed to practice in them.

Independent nurse practitioners establish their own practice in a community in order to give health services to clients who contract for this service. Nurse practitioners acquire advanced skills in physical assessment and are generally prepared at the master's degree level.

These nurses have their own group of clients that they care for in the community. They may participate in such areas as health teaching, health assessments, physical care within the realm of nursing practice, and work closely with a specific physician for the purpose of patient referral and follow-up after medical treatment has been initiated.

Psychiatric nursing, sometimes called psychiatric–mental health nursing, provides nurses with the opportunity to contribute to the care of mentally ill people and to the promotion of mental health. The setting may be a mental health clinic, a psychiatric hospital, or a psychiatric unit within a general hospital. The primary skills needed in this type of nursing are interpersonal, as the nurse must be able to recognize and deal with the complexities of relationships between individuals and within groups. Nurses, psychiatrists, social workers, and others often work in a team effort to help the mentally ill patient. Psychiatric nurses build on their basic educational base by adding clinical experiences and by participating in various forms of continuing education experiences to become increasingly expert in this field.

Community health nursing, often referred to as public health nursing, is part of the community's effort to meet the health needs of large groups of people. This area of nursing practice helps in meeting the health needs of individuals and families in their normal environment, for example, the home, school, or place of employment. The goal of this area of nursing is common to all nursing, in that the community health nurse strives to help people maintain the highest possible level of health. This is achieved by promoting and teaching good health habits, working to prevent disease, and caring for and assisting in the rehabilitation of the sick and disabled. Many times the community health nurse works in cooperation with the family in securing services from or acting as a liaison with other professionals in health, education, and social work. There are a number of programs for advanced preparation as well as numerous workshops and conferences that pertain to the specific needs of public health nurses to better prepare them to handle the responsibilities of this field.

As members of the health care team, nurses work with many other health professionals. These include such personnel as occupational therapists, physical therapists, pharmacists, dietitians, and medical technologists. In circumstances where some of these professionals are not available and patients have need of their services, nurses may be expected to expand their technical skills to fill the gap. The only health team member with whom the nurse collaborates constantly is the physician. As health care becomes more and more complex, the nurse is becoming increasingly responsible for decisions that directly influence the well-being of patients.

The registered nurse not only works with people from other fields but also directs other nursing personnel who assist in giving direct patient care. These nursing team members include practical nurses, nurse aides, and orderlies or attendants. These individuals have training that ranges from the one-year course in practical nursing that qualifies the graduate to be examined for licensure to the on-the-job training of the nurse aides and attendants.

Continuing education as well as experience are essential for nurses who wish to develop and maintain a high degree of proficiency in their field. In other words, it is frequently through the process of gaining experience, reading the literature, and enrolling in workshops and conferences that nurses may gain the knowledge and skills necessary to function in specific settings such as coronary care, intensive care, pediatrics, and geriatrics, to name only a few. Although basic skills are determined by the programs from which nurses graduate, competence and expertise develop through continuing education and experience in a given clinical setting.

The areas just discussed should not be confused with nurse anesthesiology and nurse-midwifery, two specialties that require additional education and for which certification is granted. These specialties are discussed later in this chapter.

EMPLOYMENT STATUS OF NURSES

It is common knowledge that the need for health care professionals is expanding. Nurses are no exception. Approximately half of all professional people in health care occupations today are nurses. In 1972 a total of 778,470 nurses were actively employed in the United States, as compared with 689,000 in 1968.

The ratio of nurses to state population ranges from 649 per 100,000 population in Massachusetts to 190 per 100,000 population in Arkansas, with an overall average of 390 per 100,000 population in 1973. This is an increase from 335 per 100,000 population in 1968. There has been a substantial increase in the number of registered nurses remaining in the labor force. This is probably due to a marked rise in registered nurses' salaries and to general economic conditions. There may be marked shortages of nurses in given geographical areas and a small demand for nurses in other locales.

The salary scale for registered nurses varies according to geographical location, educational background, and the type of employing agency. In 1972 most beginning practitioners earned an initial salary of $7,000 to $9,000 per year with an average annual salary of $8,200. The economic status of nursing seems to have improved as the status of women has become a more major issue in our society.

Today nursing is a flexible, far-reaching field that allows one to serve others in a variety of settings. There is a high degree of job security because of the continued need, and work opportunities are available in most geographical locations.

Nurse anesthesiology
Thelma Lang

Nurse anesthetists are registered nurses whose advanced education and training qualify them to select and administer anesthesia. They are members of the operating room team whose principal concern is maintaining the life processes of surgical patients, thus aiding surgeons in their work and contributing to the comfort and welfare of the patient.

PROFESSIONAL DEVELOPMENT

During the last two decades of the nineteenth century, surgeons in Pennsylvania and Illinois began training nurses to administer chloroform and ether. This practice spread rapidly throughout the Midwest. By 1906 the total number of cases reported in which anesthesia had been used effectively by nurse anesthetists was 14,000.

During World War I the demand for anesthetists increased the need for training programs. The Army and Navy began training nurses as anesthetists, and many of them were active in ambulance corps and in base hospital units. American nurse anesthetists trained not only other American nurses in the field but some British nurses as well.

The number of schools of anesthesia increased in the 1920s, the local and state meetings of nurse anesthetists were organized, some of them based on groups of training program alumni. In 1931 the organizational meeting for the American Association of Nurse Anesthetists (AANA) was held in Cleveland, Ohio.

When schools of anesthesia were evaluated on the basis of the criteria they used to determine their graduates' eligibility to take the qualifying examination, the need for an accreditation program became apparent. In 1946 an approval committe was established, and in 1952 the Board of Trustees of the AANA accepted the accreditation program recommended by this committee. Schools of anesthesia were notified of the minimum requirements for accreditation and were given one year to make any necessary adjustments. Revised minimum requirements adopted in 1962 included a training period of 18 months, 450 clinical cases with a total of 600 hours of clinical instruction, and 300 hours of class instruction.

The qualifying examination, first administered in 1945, is now given at more than thirty testing centers throughout the United States, and is administered by special arrangement in foreign countries. The number of schools training nurse anesthetists has increased from the fewer than 30 programs known to be in operation in the early 1920s to 201 in 1974.

RESPONSIBILITIES

Nurse anesthetists are primarily responsible for administering a prescribed anesthetic to a patient in the presence of and in accordance with the directions of either the surgeon in charge or the anesthesiologist. Their total responsibility is much more encompassing and includes an obligation to the patient, the surgeon, and to the operating room team.

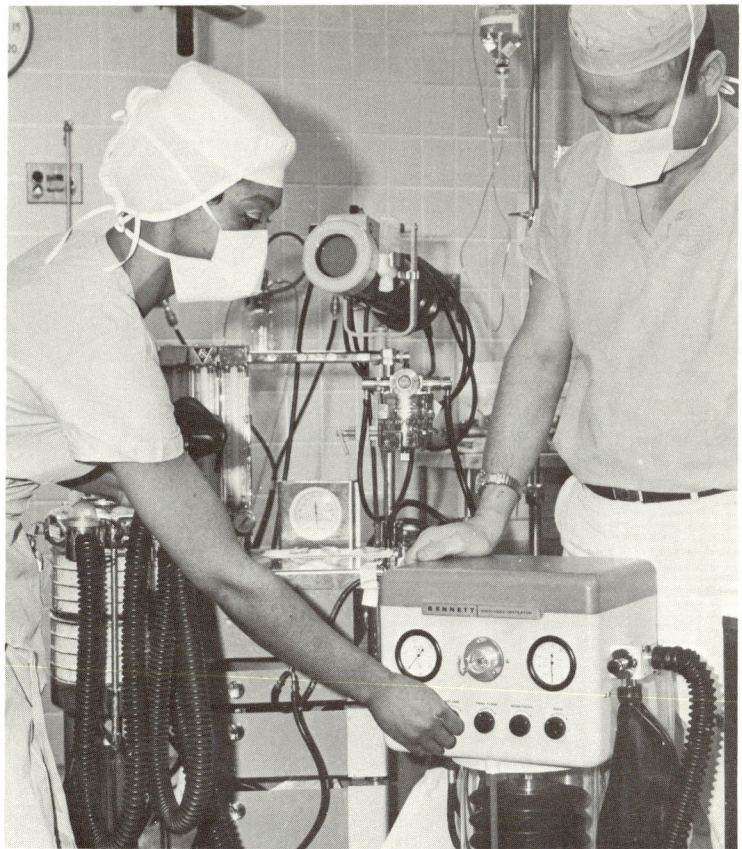

Fig. 21. It is important that all equipment be carefully prepared and checked out before an anesthetic is administered to the patient. A student nurse anesthetist, under the watchful eye of a supervisor, prepares machinery to be used during neurosurgery.

Competence in administering anesthesia to the patient requires constant alertness and good judgment, and anesthetists must refrain from any acts that can adversely affect their competence. Nurse anesthetists, like other members of the surgical team, are personally liable for their actions, regardless of whether the surgeon may be jointly or primarily liable. They should hold in confidence all information of a professional or private nature.

Nurse anesthetists must earn the physician's confidence in their ability to competently and safely administer anesthesia to the patient. It is the anesthetist's duty to give the physician the sense of security that comes with knowing that the patient is in good hands.

The nurse anesthetist must make an effort to acquire and maintain the cooperation of the operating room personnel. Any problems should be explained to the operating room nurses so that the entire surgical team can work together. The anesthetist is part of a team, and it takes the concerted efforts of each team member—physician, anesthetist, and operating room nurse—to give the patient appropriate care. (See Fig. 21.)

Nurse anesthetists have a responsibility to continue learning throughout their professional lives. Membership in the AANA is an important means of accomplishing this because it provides a method of keeping abreast of new developments and trends in the profession.

EDUCATIONAL REQUIREMENTS

Standards for evaluating the qualifications of nurse anesthetists have been established by the AANA. An applicant must be a registered nurse before entering an accredited school of anesthesia. It is recommended that the applicant have had experience in patient monitoring, as in an intensive care unit, operating room, or recovery room. An additional quarter or semester of chemistry is also suggested. The course of study, approximately eighteen months in length, includes such areas as the anatomy and physiology of the nervous, respiratory, circulatory, endocrine, and excretory systems. The physics of gases and the application of gas laws in equipment as well as methods and techniques for administering anesthetic agents are studied. The student must acquire a thorough understanding of ventilation and resuscitation, the pharmacology of anesthetic drugs, and the electronics of monitoring devices. Knowledge of these fundamental areas coupled with extensive clinical experience prepares the student for the qualifying examination. Satisfactory performance on this examination is a prerequisite for membership in the AANA. The salary for these specialists ranges from $800 to $1,500 monthly.

PERSONAL QUALITIES

Ideal nurse anesthetists are well-adjusted individuals, exhibiting high moral, professional, and ethical standards in their relationships with patients, co-workers, and employers. They approach the demands of anesthesia with skill based on knowledge and practice, and they possess inquiring minds that lead toward even higher levels of conduct and ability.

Nurse-midwifery
Ethelrine Shaw

The nurse-midwife is a registered nurse who has specialized in the care of mothers, infants, and families throughout the maternity cycle. The focus of care before, during, and after birth, as well as during the newborn and infancy periods, is the maintenance of the health and well-being of mother and child. Physical and emotional support are given not only during this process of childbearing but also through the childrearing years. The nurse-midwife is responsible for the management of clients whose condition is defined as normal according to standards established by the American College of Nurse-Midwives, the licensure laws within the state in which the nurse-midwife functions, and the definitions of normal circumstances within the agency of employment. Clients with conditions judged to be abnormal or complicated are referred to physicians.

DEVELOPMENT OF NURSE-MIDWIFERY

The practice of nurse-midwifery has matured during the twentieth century. The stereotyped image that was projected in the early 1900s by the attendant who was not educationally prepared is no longer valid. During the first decade of the twentieth century, maternity care was generally poor, regardless of who gave that care. Although training for midwives existed at that time and some nurses became midwives, it was not until 1932 that the first school for the educational preparation of nurse-midwives was established. It was called the Lobenstine Clinic, which later became the Maternity Center Association School in New York City.

In 1925 the Frontier Nursing Service was established by Mary Breckenridge in Wendover, Kentucky. This agency provided urgently needed nursing services to the hill people of Appalachia, who frequently could only be reached by horseback. The skills of nurse-midwives were well demonstrated in this population and demand for their services grew.

The services of nurse-midwives are now being endorsed by the American College of Obstetricians and Gynecologists, and salaries for these specialists range from $13,000 to $18,000 annually.

EDUCATIONAL PROGRAMS

There are two types of educational programs in nurse-midwifery. The certificate-based program provides a curriculum combining theory and clinical experience covering the entire maternity cycle. The length of the program is generally six to eight months. The master's program

Chapter 14

Occupational therapy

J. Scott Worley

The goals of occupational therapy are to promote health, prevent disability, evaluate behavior, and treat or teach individuals with psychosocial or physical dysfunction. Occupational therapy enables people to improve their ability to function in their daily lives and contributes to their sense of worth. It uses the individual's ability to accomplish tasks that are important and meaningful both as a means of evaluating abilities and of promoting active participation in health or recovery. Two essential features of occupational therapy are the therapist's analytical selection of the task to meet specific health needs of the client and the client's active participation.

DEVELOPMENT OF THE PROFESSION

The beneficial effects of physical and mental activity (occupation) have long been recognized. It was not until this century, however, that selected activivites were used to reduce the effects of illness by meeting the specific needs of an individual patient. During World War I, occupational therapists trained in the United States were sent to assist soldiers who had been wounded and were convalescing in Europe. This was the beginning of occupational therapy as it is known today. The many soldiers wounded or otherwise disabled as a result of World War II required more skilled assistance, as the advanced surgical and other lifesaving techniques meant that a great number of physically and emotionally disabled soldiers were in need of advanced rehabilitation techniques. This demand provided additional stimulus for the growth of occupational therapy. The early hospital-based training programs gave way to baccalaureate education in colleges and universities. More programs developed at the graduate level to meet the increased need for therapists with specialty skills. At present the profession is establishing itself as a community-based service through its emphasis on preventing dysfunction and maintaining health throughout an individual's life span.

PROFESSIONAL FUNCTIONS

Occupational therapy is a profession concerned with helping patients to achieve optimal development of their physical and emotional abilities. In their work, occupational therapists evaluate each patient's

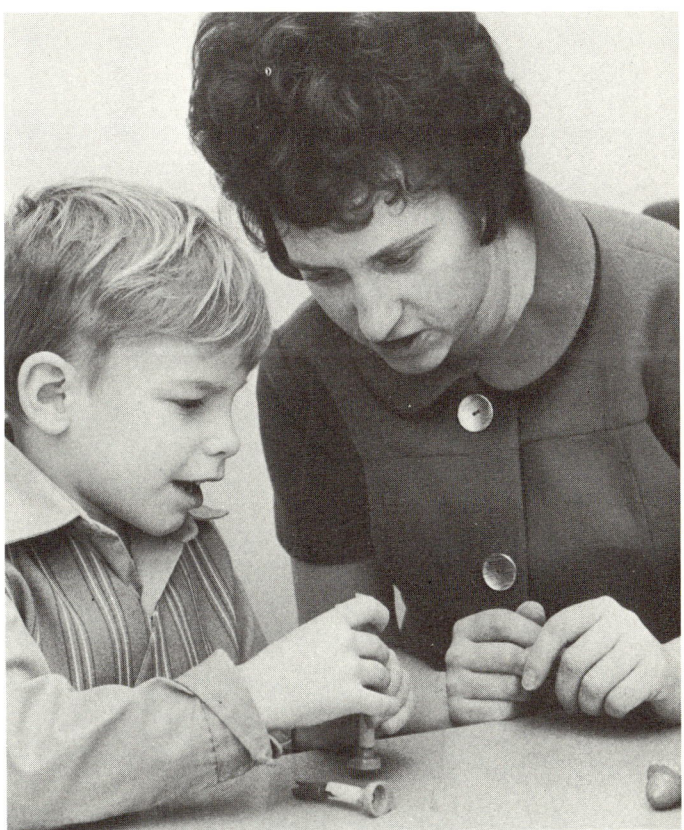

Fig. 22. Occupational therapist guides hyperkinetic child in assembling a toy manikin to aid in developing eye-hand coordination and perceptual skills.

particular physical and psychological needs and capacities and then develop an appropriate treatment program. They then determine the therapeutic attitudes and techniques necessary to help the patient. (See Fig. 22.) An understanding of medical information and human behavior, keen and perceptive observation, and recognition of individual needs make it possible for an occupational therapist to build a cooperative relationship in which both therapist and patient strive to attain the patient's highest level of performance. Therapists must discover which of the patient's specific physical and emotional needs are amenable to treatment through activity, and they must understand the meaning and dynamics of specific tasks from the cultural standpoint as well as from the perspective of the individual patient. These tasks are frequently those that are a part of the patient's normal daily life.

106 Introduction to health professions

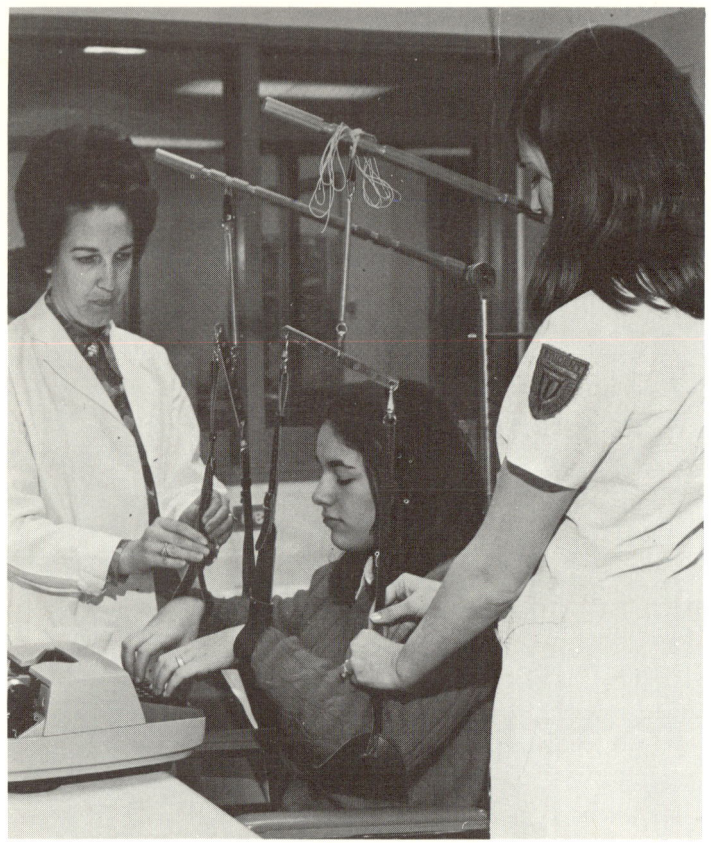

Fig. 23. A patient with partial paralysis of the arms is evaluated to determine if slings or other supports will allow her to type.

The occupational therapist works with patients individually and in groups, using a variety of creative, educational, industrial, manual, musical, prevocational, and recreational activities to enhance motor function and promote psychological, social, and economic adjustment. Teaching patients to regain daily living skills through the use of artificial limbs, assistive devices, or special equipment is an additional responsibility of the therapist. (See Fig. 23.)

As a member of the professional health team, the occupational therapist plans and works cooperatively with nurses, physical therapists, and vocational counselors to help patients achieve their highest potential. The patients may be of any age and may suffer from cardiac or neurological impairment, arthritis, physical injury, mental retardation, emotional disturbance or virtually any disability. Occupational therapists

Occupational therapy   **107**

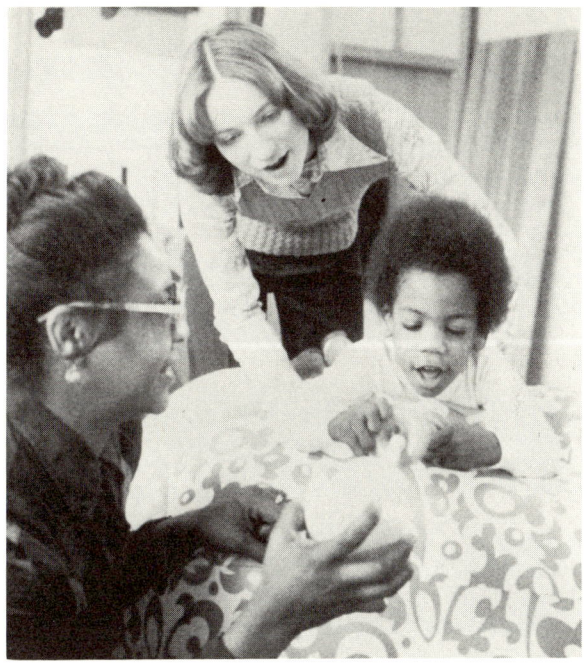

Fig. 24. A mother learns that she can help her child to use his arms and play more effectively by first properly positioning him.

work in a variety of settings, including children's hospitals, general hospitals, rehabilitation centers, psychiatric clinics, schools, sheltered workshops, services for the homebound, and other community agencies. (See Fig. 24.) Some therapists, working in conjunction with qualified professionals, establish their own practices. The following case study illustrates some of the contributions an occupational therapist can make to health care.

Janet, who is 5 years of age, participates very normally now in her kindergarten class, using her prosthetic right arm nearly as efficiently as she would have used her own hand. At the age of 2½ years, Janet was involved in an automobile accident. Her injuries resulted in the amputation of her right arm. Because of head injuries, she was unconscious for nearly a week. Her mother, who had been driving when the accident occured, also had a very difficult adjustment period afterward. Occupational therapy played an important role in both Janet's recovery and her mother's readjustment.

The occupational therapist and the aide were the first to discover the child's returning consciousness and were able to promote her first awareness of her surroundings. They had been applying various touch, sound, smell, and taste stimuli at the time Janet first showed signs of awakening. Further change of the odors presented encouraged her to regain full consciousness and enabled the hospital staff to perform procedures that had been delayed until then.

During the early stages of Janet's recovery the occupational therapist also carefully evaluated the nature of her play and used some specific tests to determine whether there were any problems of motor coordination or perception as a result of her injuries. Fortunately no problems were noted, and consequently that portion of the occupational therapy program designed to encourage Janet's normal development with play and interaction with other children was not complicated.

Even before the little girl was first fitted with a prosthesis and brought to the occupational therapy department for training in its use, her therapist had already made important contributions to the prosthetic and amputee evaluation team by providing vital information about Janet's level of development at play and in other activities. The therapist had also participated in deciding when the prosthesis should be provided and in selecting the type of prosthesis to be used.

When she began to work with her occupational therapist, Janet quickly learned to use the device as a part of the daily play and self-care activities that the therapist had specifically designed for training purposes. She had no difficulty in learning to use subsequent prostheses that were prescribed as she grew. The occupational therapist checked out the mechanical and functional efficiency of each new prosthesis, and when Janet received the last one, she suggested an adjustment in the placement of a strap so Janet could put on the prosthesis more easily by herself. During this period the therapist was in close contact with Janet's family, suggesting toys and play activities that were appropriate for her level of interest as a growing, active child and that would also help her to develop more skill in using her prothesis in self-care.

Janet's mother had not been physically injured in the accident, but because she had been driving the car, she was initially unable to adjust emotionally and held herself responsible for her daughter's injuries. She therefore received psychiatric help on an outpatient basis, and occupational therapy was part of her treatment. In that setting the occupational therapist's evaluation of how Janet's mother dealt with the tasks provided and with the other people in the treatment setting was used extensively in conjunction with specific evaluative procedures to guide further treatment. The ability of Janet's mother to function in her daily relationships was assessed on the basis of her response in these situations. The tasks and group situations in occupational therapy were carefully controlled and provided Janet's mother with an opportunity to handle her feelings of guilt, depression, and worthlessness. This treatment facilitated her eventual discharge from the outpatient program.

Close communication was maintained between the two therapists working with Janet and her mother in order to prevent complications and facilitate the treatment of both mother and daughter.

Even though she is now doing well in kindergarten, Janet will probably be receiving occupational therapy in the future. Each time she needs a larger prosthesis, occupational therapy will make a contribution, and hopefully complications and adjustment problems will be minimal as she grows through adolescence into adulthood.

PERSONNEL AND EDUCATION

Registered occupational therapists (O.T.R.) are professionally qualified graduates of occupational therapy programs that are accredited by the American Medical Association in collaboration with the American Occupational Therapy Association (AOTA). They have successfully completed the national certifying examination and maintain registered membership in the AOTA. The therapist functions at a level that may involve supervision, administration, and consultation in addition to the evaluation, planning, and execution of treatment programs. The roles assumed by individual therapists depend on their qualifications, areas of competence, and interests.

Educational requirements of occupational therapy curricula are geared to fulfilling the requirements for program accreditation. In addition to meeting certain specified minimum standards, each approved program must provide instruction in the basic human sciences, the human development process, specific life tasks and activities (their various implications and analysis), the health-illness-health continuum, and the principles, theory, and application of occupation therapy. In addition, each program must meet the requirements of the university in which it is offered and must provide a minimum of six months of field experience.

Professional qualification (registration) may be obtained in one of four ways. First, students may enroll at a college or university that offers an accredited occupational therapy program at the baccalaureate level. A second approach may be through occupational therapy curricula offering eighteen-to twenty-two-month programs for college graduates who have received baccalaureate degrees in related fields. There are a limited number of these programs, and they provide a certificate in occupational therapy, making those who complete the course eligible to take the national certifying examination. These curriculums should not be confused with the programs for certified occupational therapy assistants that are described later in this section. The third approach involves basic preparation in occupational therapy at the graduate level. The number of these programs is increasing, and they offer masters' degrees in occupational therapy for persons with undergraduate majors in biology, psychology, sociology, or other fields related to occupational therapy.

The fourth method permits technically qualified persons (for example, a C.O.T.A., see p. 110) to seek registration as professional occupational therapists. They may become eligible to take the AOTA examination for registration after completing two years of work experience under the supervision of a registered occupational therapist

(O.T.R.) and certification that they have successfully completed the required six-month field experience.

After achieving eligibility by one of these four methods and after successful completion of six months of field experience under the supervision of a qualified supervisor, candidates may take the examination for registration by the AOTA.

There are an increasing number of graduate programs designed to permit registered occupational therapists to do advanced work in preparation for specialized clinical practice, research, or teaching in occupational therapy programs. These programs offer degrees at both the master's and doctoral levels.

Certified occupational therapy assistants (C.O.T.A.) function under the supervision of a registered occupational therapist in general activity, maintenance, and supportive programs of specific treatment. To become certified by the AOTA, it is necessary to complete an AOTA-approved technical training program and meet certification requirements.

These training programs include (1) studies of normal human structure, function, growth, and development; (2) studies of illness and injury and their effects on the patient; (3) experience with a variety of media used in occupational therapy; (4) principles and practice of occupational therapy; and (5) practical experience supervised by a registered occupational therapist.

Programs may vary in length from twenty-one weeks to two years, depending on the type of program and its location. Two-year associate degree programs are offered by an increasing number of junior colleges. Graduates who meet the requirements may pass the examination and be employed as certified occupational therapy assistants or they may receive some credit for transfer to a professional program at the baccalaureate level. Programs are also sponsored by the military services, vocational and technical schools, and public school departments of adult education.

Some programs may restrict admission to people from a particular geographical area or have a employment requirement for admission. Therefore those who are interested in becoming certified occupational therapy assistants should check the requirements of specific programs.

Occupational therapy aides are trained on the job to meet the requirements and standards of the occupational therapy departments in which they work. They are directed or supervised by a registered therapist or certified occupational therapy assistant and may perform clerical, maintenance, or patient-related duties.

PROFESSIONAL ORGANIZATION

The American Occupational Therapy Association is the national organization of occupational therapists, and participation involves the professional, technical, and student levels of personnel within the profession. It is composed of local organizations (usually at the state level) that are affiliated with it and have representation in its policymaking body. The AOTA establishes standards within the profession and provides means of communication within the profession through newsletters and journals. The AOTA's goal is to foster educational and professional growth in the practice of occupational therapy for the improvement of the public's health.

PROFESSIONAL OPPORTUNITIES

There are not enough occupational therapists to fill all the positions available each year both in this country and abroad. In addition to direct contact with patients through treatment, therapists may be involved in research, teaching, consultation, and administration. The increasing national emphasis on health has opened many new frontiers of service, creating virtually limitless opportunities in this exciting and challenging profession.

In general, salary opportunities compare favorably with those of other health-related professions with comparable qualifying requirements. With specialty experience, experience in supervision or administration, or additional educational background, therapists may assume additional responsibilities and may receive appropriately higher salaries.

SUGGESTED READINGS

American Journal of Occupational Therapy, published monthly by American Occupational Therapy Association.

Description of function in occupational therapy, New York, no date, American Occupational Therapy Association.

History of occupational therapy, American Journal of Occupational Therapy **21**(5): entire issue, 1967.

Reference Manual for Occupational Therapy Educators, Rockville, Md., 1974, American Occupational Therapy Association.

Reilly, M.: Occupational therapy can be one of the great ideas of 20th century medicine, American Journal of Occupational Therapy **16**:1, 1962.

Spackman, C. S.: A history of the practice of occupational therapy for the restoration of function for the physically disabled, American Journal of Occupational Therapy **22**:67, 1968

The A-B-C's of occupational therapy, Greenfield, Mass., 1969, Channing L. Bete Co., Inc.

West, W.: Statement to the Committee on Health Manpower, American Journal of Occupational Therapy **22**:89, 1968.

Yerxa, E.: Authentic occupational therapy, American Journal of Occupational Therapy **21**:1, 1967.

PROFESSIONAL ORGANIZATION WHERE FURTHER INFORMATION CAN BE OBTAINED

American Occupational Therapy Association
6000 Executive Boulevard
Rockville, Maryland 20852

Chapter 15
Optometry
James F. Noe

Optometry is the health profession specializing in the care of people's vision. Although modern optometry is a relatively young profession, its earliest foundations can be traced back to the Middle Ages. Like the other major health professions, optometry owes its present stature to a number of scientific discoveries and a series of contributing scientists.

PROFESSIONAL DEVELOPMENT

Visual care prior to 1300 A.D. was practically nonexistent. Spectacles had not been invented, and visual defects were merely tolerated. People suffering from "dimness of the eyes" were primarily thought to have an eye disease. They were considered to be useless members of society and were treated accordingly.

During the period between 1300 and 1900, astronomers, mathematicians, physicists, and other physical scientists made important contributions to the understanding of vision and the science of optics. Spectacle lenses were developed, and a limited number of people in the more technologically advanced nations were able to procure some primitive correction for their visual difficulties.

Additional optical knowledge and the development of modern physiological optics led to the era of "modern optometry." The first training school for optometrists in the United States was established in 1892, and in 1901 the first state optometry licensing law was passed. The remainder of the states passed licensing laws in rapid succession, and the profession continued to develop.

Formation of state and national professional organizations, the increased number and quality of optometric training institutions, and the growing demand for and acceptance of professional optometric services served to enhance the growth of optometry as a vital health care profession.

PROFESSIONAL FUNCTIONS

Optometrist today offer a variety of professional services. They provide comprehensive assistance to the public in maintaining and enhancing good vision and correcting vision defects. Their work involves much more than merely correcting blurred vision, although this is an extremely important function. A number of diagnostic tests are per-

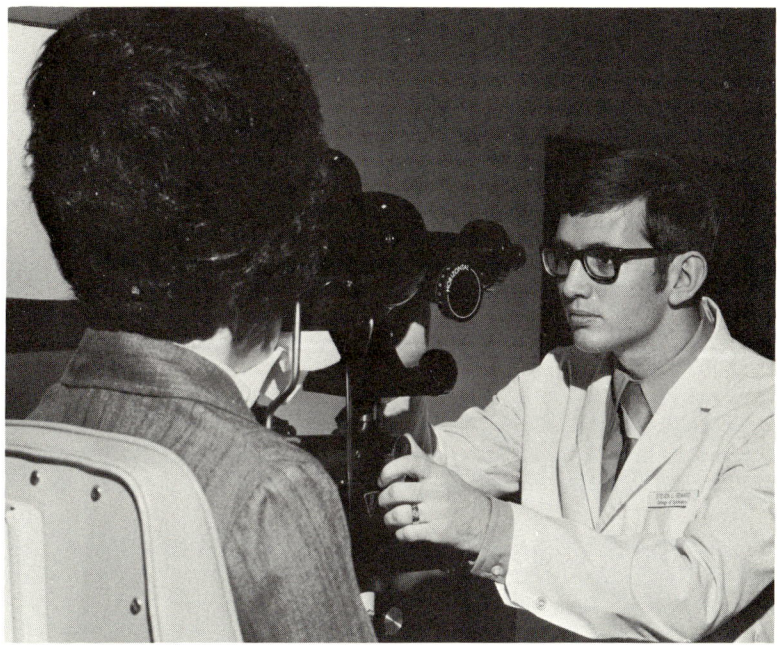

Fig. 25. One of a series of diagnostic tests is administered to determine the health and efficiency of the visual system.

formed by the optometrist to determine how the eyes of the patient focus and adjust to critical near and far distances. (See Fig. 25.) The eyes are a complex system, and people require different types of visual abilities to read a textbook, drive an automobile, pilot an airplane, or enjoy a movie or television.

It often takes an optometrist many hours over a number of months to provide the necessary services demanded even in routine cases. This health care professional is much more than a mere provider of eyeglasses. The optometrist must provide basic optometric services for every patient. The eyes must be carefully examined for possible disease conditions. This requires the expert use of a number of scientific instruments and an applied knowledge of anatomy, physiology, and pathology.

Vision must be scientifically measured and a determination made of the patient's ability to use his eyes to see, focus, and aim with accuracy and comfort. These measurements and findings must then be carefully analyzed to ensure the most efficient solution to any vision problem that has been detected.

An exact set of instructions has to be prepared so that the scientific and technical compounding of any corrective materials can be made by the laboratory. This finished prescription must then be carefully adjusted to the eyes of the individual patient to ensure maximum results as well as comfort.

More complex cases call for more complicated testing. Problems in color vision, image-size measurements, binocular (or two-eyed) coordination, fields of vision, and depth perception are some of the more involved areas that demand careful testing by trained optometrists. Each of these areas requires specialized training, techniques, and equipment to reach accurate solutions to the patient's problems.

Many times it will be determined that prescription glasses are not necessary to solve a particular problem. The optometrist may prescribe visual training or orthoptics to remedy the diagnosed visual defect. These eye exercises must be carefully planned and explained to the patient to maximize their effectiveness. Often the optometrist will assist the patient in this treatment, using special scientific apparatus over an extended period of time. Such conditions as crossed eyes in children often lend themselves to this type of corrective measure.

Older patients present a different type of challenge to the optometrist. Correction of their visual problems often requires more than a single lens prescription. Specially designed bifocals, trifocals, or quadrifocals must be carefully prescribed to deal effectively with the needs of these patients.

The specialty of fitting contact lenses occupies a large segment of many optometrists' practices. The intricate measurements and careful fitting techniques required by this optometric service are challenging and time consuming. Constant practice, study, and education are required to keep abreast of the latest developments. Ever-increasing numbers of people are selecting this type of visual correction, and the optometrist has the responsibility of keeping up-to-date in this rapidly changing area of specialization.

CAREERS IN OPTOMETRY

Most optometrists enter private practice. A majority of private practices have traditionally consisted of an individual optometrist assisted by one or more optometric aides. However, the present trend seems to be toward practices in which several optometrists with different areas of interest form a group practice, each contributing to a comprehensive optometric service.

There are various areas of specialization within optometry, in addition to the fitting of contact lenses. These include the examination and optical rehabilitation of aniseikonia, a discrepancy in the size of the images seen by each of the two eyes; the diagnosis and rehabilitation of problems involving binocular coordination and visual perception; the analysis and solution of visual problems associated with aviation, automobile driving, and other forms of transportation and with industry and schoolwoork; and the correction of partial or subnormal vision. The goal is to help achieve clear, comfortable, safe, and efficient vision not only by optical means but also by making recommendations for enhancing the visual environment through better illumination, improved visibility of objects, and better design of equipment.

Optometrists are also employed by hospitals and clinics and by federal, state, and local agencies. A sizable number of optometrists serve as optometry officers in the Army, Navy, or Air Force or in the United States Public Health Service. Currently, graduate optometrists enter the Army and Air Force with the rank of captain and enter the Navy as lieutenants, junior grade.

Industry and government also employ optometrists in various research and development areas. For example, optometrists are involved in the National Aeronautics and Space Administration programs and in the work of major aviation companies as well as in the research projects of the larger optical manufacturing companies.

Optometrists are also needed to teach in colleges of optometry. Many of the colleges offer graduate programs in physiological optics for those optometrists interested in careers in education or research.

PERSONAL QUALITIES

Both men and women find optometry a rewarding career. An aptitude for and interest in science and mathematics coupled with a desire to be of service to people are the characteristics most important to an aspiring optometrist.

The personal satisfaction derived from rendering an important service combined with an adequate income make optometry an appealing health profession. Optometrists can determine their own office hours to best suit the requirements of patients and family. Women optometrists find this flexibility especially attractive in combining a career with marriage.

The income of optometrists depends on their professional skills and the services they provide. Their income should equal that of the other professional men in their chosen community. Recent reports cite an average net income in excess of $20,000 per year for the established practitioner.

EDUCATIONAL PREPARATION

Present educational requirements for the profession consist of a four-year optometric curriculum preceded by a minimum of two years of specific preoptometry study. This preoptometry work can be completed at any accredited college or university, but the four-year professional training can be pursued only at one of the institutions accredited by the Council on Optometric Education of the American Optometic Association (AOA). There are presently twelve accredited schools of optometry located in the population centers of the United States. Three additional schools are scheduled to begin admitting students in the near future.

Academic preparation for optometry should begin in high school with a college preparatory program in English, social studies, mathematics, science, and foreign language. Preoptometry curriculums include courses in chemistry, physics, biology, psychology, and mathematics. Professional curriculums embrace the various facets of the profession and include ocular anatomy, optics, psychology, and both the theory and practical application of optometric techniques. Students also spend a large part of their professional training in clinical settings. Under the supervision of the clinical staff, students work with patients to learn and refine the various skills so important in their future practices.

On successful completion of the professional curriculum, a student receives the Doctor of Optometry (O.D.) degree, which makes him eligible to take the state board examination required in every state for licensure to practice optometry.

OPTOMETRIC ASSISTANTS

The optometrist's role has been refined in recent years by the addition of auxiliary personnel in the area of clinical practice. Although exact job descriptions vary according to the size of the optometric practice and the type of services provided by the doctor, these assistants share certain general responsibilities.

Most optometrists employ an optometric office assistant who serves as receptionist, office manager, and housekeeper. An assistant's main tasks are scheduling daily appointments, preparing and filing patient examination records, billing, receiving fees, and attending to the details of operating an efficiently run professional office.

Most office assistants receive on-the-job training and their role is determined by their education and former experience. In addition, many optometrists encourage their assistants to attend periodic workshops and seminars sponsored by local and state optometry associations. These are often held in conjunction with state conventions and afford an opportunity for assistants to update their knowledge of optometry office management, meet other assistants, and exchange ideas and procedures with them.

As an optometrist's practice grows, he may wish to employ an assistant to perform some of the more routine optometric tests. These assistants are referred to as optometric technicians, and their specific functions are determined by their education and experience in the area of optometry. The optometrist for whom the technician works carefully determines which diagnostic tests the technician can perform for a given patient to ensure an accurate vision analysis and diagnosis. These tests may differ from one patient to another and often need to be carefully supervised and validated by the optometrist.

A more exacting description of the optometric technician's role is presently being evolved, and training programs for technicians are being developed at a number of optometry schools and other institutions of higher education that specialize in the preparation of health care technicians. With the growing demand for more efficient health care at all levels for a rapidly increasing population, the optometric technician seems to be one answer to the problem of the shortage of optometrists in the United States.

FUTURE OUTLOOK

The complex demands made on vision by modern-day living create a steadily increasing demand for optometric services. As our population increases, so does the need for greater numbers of professionals in all areas of health care.

Numerous studies indicate that at present the 19,000 optometrists in the United States are not able to meet even the current need for services. Estimates of future needs are as high as an additional 1,000 graduates per year for the decade of the 1970s. Even with the newer methods of health care delivery being planned, there remains a critical need in all health professions for well-qualified, highly motivated men and women.

SUMMARY

Optometry as a profession has had a relatively short history. With the various services optometrists are now able to offer, the profession is beginning to realize its full potential as a part of the health care system. It is striving to meet the challenges of our growing population and the ever-increasing demand for quality health services. It offers a unique challenge to the student searching for a way to make a meaningful contribution to our complex society.

REFERENCES

Gregg, J. R.: Your future in optometry, New York, 1968, Richards Rosen Press.

Hirsch, M. J., and Wick, R. E.: The optometric profession, Philadelphia, 1968, Chilton Book Co.

Kitchell, F.: Opportunities in an optometry career, New York, 1967, Universal Publishing & Distributing Co.

PROFESSIONAL ORGANIZATION WHERE FURTHER INFORMATION CAN BE OBTAINED

American Optometric Association
Vocational Guidance Department
7000 Chippewa Street
St. Louis, Missouri 63119

Chapter 16
Pharmacy
David A. Knapp and James A. Visconti

Pharmacists are the most accessible of all American health workers. The pharmacy, their place of practice, may be found on almost any corner of any street in the country, and it has become a modern American institution. However, pharmacy is one of the most ancient of the professions. Since the dawn of history there have been those who have dedicated themselves to the development of drugs for healing and comforting the sick. Written prescriptions have been found that date from as early as 3600 B.C., and the Ebers papyrus, written about 1550 B.C., contains references to many chemicals, formulas, and cosmetics used at that time. In these years the professions of medicine and pharmacy were as one, and it was not until the Arabian period (700 to 1000 A.D.) that pharmacy was first delineated as a separate profession.

In America, pharmacists have always served as a necessary adjunct to the nation's physicians. Prior to the industrial revolution they personally compounded and prepared a large proportion of the remedies used in the practice of medicine. With the growth of pharmaceutical manufacturing, the technical work of compounding has been markedly reduced in the practice of the community pharmacist, although pharmacists continue to perform this vital function when necessary.

Today, nearly everyone is familiar with the pharmacist's major professional task—that of compounding and dispensing medications for individual patients. Not everyone is aware, however, of the knowledge and responsibility involved in performing this deceptively simple task. With the increasing number and sophistication of medicinal agents now available to combat disease, it has become even more important to have a highly trained health professional responsible for the safe and effective use of these products. The pharmacist is such a person.

There are presently about 132,000 pharmacists in the United States. About 108,000 practice in community settings, another 13,300 work in hospitals, and there are approximately 10,400 in academic or industrial settings. There is presently a great demand for pharmacists, since prescription volume has been increasing steadily at a rate of about 10% a year for almost the last 10 years. This rate of increase should continue for some years to come, especially with the advent of government-supported health programs such as Medicare that have expanded the market for drugs and will no doubt eventually provide for outpatient prescription services as well as drugs for inpatients.

COMMUNITY PHARMACISTS AND PRESCRIPTION DRUGS

Most of today's pharmacists are employed in community or neighborhood pharmacies. They come into contact with literally hundreds of patients each week and dispense over 1.4 billion prescriptions a year. Each of those prescriptions represents an explicit order for a specific kind of drug for an individual patient. It is the responsibility of the pharmacist to determine whether the prescription includes the correct dosage, whether it will be compatible with other medications that the patient may be taking, and whether the directions for use are clear and complete. After selecting or preparing the proper drug and dosage form, the pharmacist must be sure that the medication is packaged in the right container and that the patient understands how to use it. For complete pharmaceutical service this usually requires a face-to-face discussion of the medication with the individual patient.

Obviously even the best of our modern drugs will be of no value if taken improperly or not at all. For example, many people think that a liquid antibiotic preparation for a baby's earache should be dripped directly into the ear rather than given orally. Some medications cause a patient's urine to change color, and unless he is told to expect this, a frantic call to the physician may result. A number of widely prescribed antibiotics are not absorbed properly if they are taken with milk. Since these products are often prescribed for children, a parent may give the child the capsule with a glass of milk, thus reducing the effectiveness of the therapy.

The pharmacist must also be alert to the possibility of drug interactions. With today's sophisticated drug therapy, it is not uncommon for a patient to be taking several drugs simultaneously, and some of these may interact with each other to the detriment of his health. Many patients today are under the care of several different physicians, and consequently a patient may receive prescriptions for the same drug from each. This is frequently the case with tranquilizers, since they are prescribed commonly by different kinds of specialists in medicine. Thus it is sometimes possible for a patient to be taking double or even triple the appropriate dosage of a particular drug, and this can sometimes result in dangerous overdoses. This type of problem is difficult to detect unless accurate drug histories of individual patients are kept. Many modern pharmacists are incorporating such patient prescription records into their practice. When new patients come to the pharmacist, they are asked to complete a patient record card, indicating any drug allergies or other problems that they may have. Other drugs that the patient may be taking are also recorded, so that every time a prescription is dispensed at that particular pharmacy, the patient's record card can be checked to see whether there are any possibilities of drug interactions or overdoses. The biggest drawback of this system is that patients must have all of their prescriptions dispensed at one pharmacy if all drugs are to be noted on the record card. Pharmacists are now experimenting with filing patient prescription records from many pharmacies in a computer in an effort to overcome this problem. Any cooperating pharmacy could then draw needed information from the computer file through a simple telephone call.

OTHER FUNCTIONS OF COMMUNITY PHARMACISTS

Pharmacists are in a strategic position to offer substantial professional services to the patient in connection with prescription drugs. However, this is by no means the only area in which they can make a contribution. The corner pharmacy is the largest source of self-medication products in the country, and the pharmacist is readily available to offer advice and counsel on the use of such agents. American families practice self-medication on a rather large basis; in fact, the typical family spends more than $40 each year on nonprescription drugs. Although pharmacists are not trained to diagnose and prescribe drugs for medical problems, they are qualified to make comparative judgments on the quality and effectiveness of the drugs that they dispense, and they are called on to do this quite frequently in everyday practice. Pharmacists may also provide professional services to the public by stocking and distributing surgical appliances and prescription accessories.

Some community pharmacists have expanded their professional services by acting as consultants to nursing homes and extended care facilities. Such facilities are usually not able to employ a full-time pharmacist and rely on the neighborhood pharmacist to meet their pharmaceutical needs.

HOSPITAL PHARMACIES

Another major area of employment for practicing pharmacists is the hospital. In contrast to their colleagues in the community, hospital pharmacists are generally most concerned with serving the needs of inpatients at the institution, although some outpatient dispensing may be offered. In the hospital setting, pharmacists may also be responsible for such tasks as bulk compounding, the development and implementation of intravenous admixture programs, and the control of drug use within the institution. (See Fig. 26.) The hospital pharmacy often serves as a drug information center for the hospital and in some instances for the entire community. Here pharmacists, generally those who have some graduate training, analyze and compile information about drug products, including new drugs that may be available only for investigational use within the hospital.

Pharmacists in the hospital setting often come into contact with members of other health professions. For example, they may work in continuing education programs with physicians and other health workers. They may interact with the nursing staff in monitoring the drug therapy of inpatients and in attempting to minimize medication

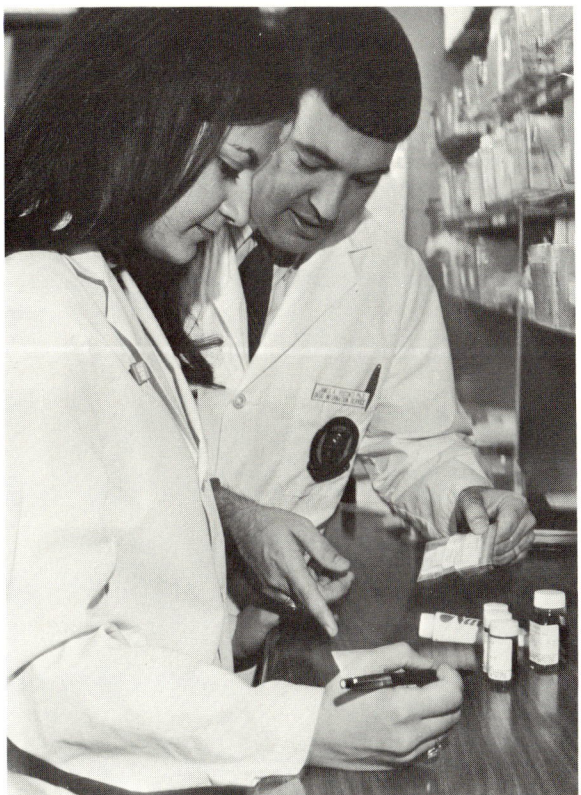

Fig. 26. A hospital pharmacist and physician discuss the choice of a patient's prescription drug.

errors. They work with the medical dietitian, paying particular attention to food-drug interactions that may affect the well-being of the patient. For example, some foods may completely inactivate certain types of drugs, as in the case of the antibiotic-milk combination mentioned previously. In other cases, certain drug-food combinations may produce severe reactions in some patients.

Pharmacists may also be called on to consult in poisoning cases, and the poison prevention centers in many hospitals are staffed by pharmacists. Drug therapy can sometimes change the normal values to be expected from certain laboratory diagnostic procedures, and therefore pharmacists and medical technologists often work closely together. Thus it is apparent that the pharmacist contributes to the well-being of the patient in the hospital in many ways beyond the mere compounding and dispensing of pharmaceuticals.

OTHER CAREER OPPORTUNITIES

Although community and hospital practices employ the largest number of pharmacy graduates, opportunities exist for pharmacists in a variety of other settings. The armed forces need pharmacists for military service, and the United States Public Health Service has opportunities in Indian health programs and federal hospitals. Pharmacists engage in health planning and administration through various federal and state agencies such as the Food and Drug Administration and state boards of pharmacy. Positions are available in the drug industry for pharmacists interested in laboratory work, drug development, and sales. Advanced degrees are generally required for research positions in industry or for teaching positions in the nation's seventy-two accredited colleges of pharmacy. It is clear that the unique training of the pharmacist provides for great flexibility in career choice on graduation.

STARTING SALARIES

The pharmacy graduate of today commands perhaps the highest starting salary of any bachelor's degree graduate in the country. Positions in community pharmacy are financially rewarding, and especially attractive salaries are available in larger cities. Hospital salaries are somewhat lower, as are those paid for positions in government and industry. Pharmacists with advanced degrees may draw larger salaries.

WOMEN IN PHARMACY

The profession of pharmacy has become increasingly attractive to women, who comprise about 27% of the students in training today. Good salaries, flexible hours, and pleasant working conditions will probably continue to attract more women to the field.

EDUCATIONAL AND PRACTICAL REQUIREMENTS

The professional program in pharmacy is five years in length, and graduates earn the degree of bachelor of science in pharmacy. The first two years consist of study in the basic sciences. These include general and organic chemistry, biology, anatomy, and physiology, physics, and mathematics. These requirements can often be met at community colleges or branch campuses of universities. The last three years must be spent in a college of pharmacy. Areas of study include pharmacognosy (the study of drugs of plant or animal origin), medicinal chemistry (the study of drugs of synthetic origin and the relation of the chemical structure of drug products to their action on the body), pharmacology (the study of the action of drug products on living systems), pharmaceutics (the study of the effect of dosage forms on drug activity), the social and administrative sciences (studies of the social, psychological, public health, and administrative aspects of the practice of pharmacy), and the clinical or professional practice area (the integration of material from the basic sciences and its applications to the practice of pharmacy).

After graduation from an accredited college of pharmacy, the aspiring pharmacist must take a licensing examination administered by the state board of pharmacy. This examination usually requires three days and includes theoretical examinations concerning the separate disciplines of the curriculum plus a practical examination. Most states require the completion of one year of intership in a pharmacy before the board examination may be taken, although some states now recognize shorter periods of externship under the supervision of a school of pharmacy. After successfully passing the examination, the candidate becomes licensed to practice pharmacy. There is reciprocity concerning licensure in some states. In others, the candidate must be reexamined.

ADVANCED EDUCATION PROGRAMS

Students who wish to pursue graduate studies in pharmacy may choose either professionally oriented or research oriented programs. Professional graduate degrees include the doctor of pharmacy and the master's degree in hospital pharmacy; both require two to three years of additional study, mainly in clinical areas. Some programs include residencies that offer practical experience in hospitals. Graduates assume positions of great responsibility in professional settings.

Research degrees at the master's and the doctor's levels are offered in each of the pharmaceutical sciences. Doctoral programs require three to five years of additional study and include a dissertation. They prepare graduates for research positions in industry or for academic positions.

SUMMARY

There is a distinct need for properly educated pharmacists in a variety of positions. Pharmacists in all areas of practice and in every geographical location share the primary responsibility of contributing to the safe and effective use of drugs by all who need them.

SUGGESTED READINGS

Deno, R. A., Rowe, T. D., and Brodie, D. C.: The profession of pharmacy, Philadelphia, 1966, J. B. Lippincott Co.

Gable, F. B.: Opportunities in pharmacy careers, New York, 1964, Universal Publishing & Distributing Corp.

Sonnedecker, G. L.: Kremers and Urdang's history of pharmacy, ed. 3, Philadelphia, 1963, J. B. Lippincott Co.

PROFESSIONAL ORGANIZATION WHERE FURTHER INFORMATION CAN BE OBTAINED

American Pharmaceutical Association
2215 Constitution Avenue, N.W.
Washington, D.C. 20037

Chapter 17
Physical therapy
Frank M. Pierson

Physical therapy is one of several health professions that has been developed and expanded to meet the needs of the citizens of the United States and the world. Physical therapy offers challenges to and provides stimulation for individuals who desire to satisfy societal and personal needs by working with people in a scientifically and medically oriented profession.

The evaluation and treatment of specific patient abilities and disabilities, both mental and physical, are two important functions of the physical therapist. (See Fig. 27.) Primary objectives of all treatment programs are to restore the individual to independent function, to maintain normal general health, and to prevent disability. Persons of all ages, economic levels, and cultural backgrounds are treated by the physical therapist in a variety of settings and environments. Treatment programs are developed and implemented on the basis of a knowledge of each patient's condition, the factors that have produced or caused it, and the factors that can correct, improve, or alleviate the problem.

A variety of exercise techniques and specific types of equipment are employed to obtain the results that will most effectively assist the patient. The selection and proper application of the most appropriate treatment procedures and equipment are also the responsibility of the physical therapist.

HISTORICAL REVIEW

The profession of physical therapy was founded during World War I by a group of women who functioned as "reconstruction aides" within the United States Army with the express purpose of promoting the physical restoration of injured service personnel. The first formally organized physical therapy department was established by the United States Army at Walter Reed Hospital in Washington, D.C., in 1916.

After World War I these women continued to utilize their skills in civilian life, and by 1921 the American Women's Therapeutic Association had been organized. In 1922 the group became known as the American Physiotherapy Association. The present organizational title, The American Physical Therapy Association (APTA), was approved in 1948.

The APTA maintains a paid and volunteer staff to assist its 19,000

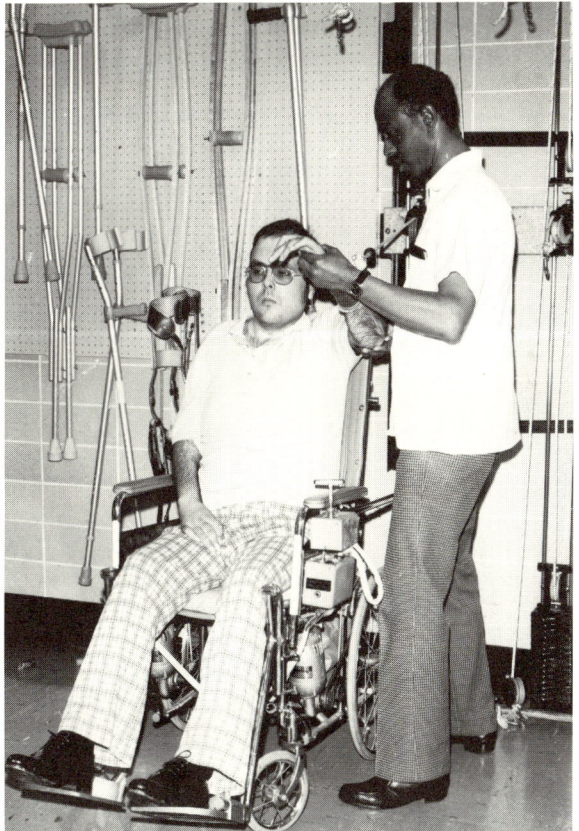

Fig. 27. A physical therapist and a man with paralysis resulting from an automobile accident work together to strengthen remaining shoulder function.

members with educational, legislative, public relations, financial, and related activities. There are fifty-three chapters of the Association in each of the fifty states, the District of Columbia, Puerto Rico, and the Virgin Islands, and most chapters are subdivided into districts. Membership in the APTA is voluntary, and it is the only organization in the United States that directly attempts to protect the general welfare of physical therapists through legislative activities, continuing education programs, professional publications, and support for the economic well-being of its members.

EDUCATIONAL PROGRAMS

Four types of physical therapy educational programs are available: associate degree, baccalaureate degree, certificate, and graduate degree.

Regardless of the type of program, each must be located in a college or university and each program must be approved and accredited by the APTA and the Council on Medical Education of the American Medical Association.

The program that terminates in a baccalaureate degree requires four years of academic preparation in an institution of higher learning, including one to two years of preprofessional course work and two to three years of professionally oriented course work. The preprofessional requirements usually include courses in the basic sciences (mathematics, physics, chemistry, etc.), the humanities (English, philosophy, fine arts, etc.), and the social sciences (psychology, sociology, history, etc.). The professional courses include study in areas of advanced natural science (physiology and anatomy), specific physical therapy courses, general medical information courses, and clinical educational experiences.

Certificate programs are available in several institutions, and enrollment is usually limited to students who have previously completed a baccalaureate degree. Prerequisite requirements for admission may include: completion of specific natural and social science course work (chemistry, physics, physiology, anatomy, sociology, psychology), evidence of satisfactory academic ability, and evidence of participation in some type of health care program. Twelve to twenty-four months may be required for completion of the academic and clinical phases of the certificate program.

In recent years, several graduate programs have been developed to provide an advanced degree in physical therapy or in allied health (medical) professions. Admission to these programs depends on the fulfillment of specific graduate school requirements and previous completion of a baccalaureate degree or certificate in physical therapy. Students occasionally are admitted as undergraduates, and on completion of an extensive academic and clinical education program, they are granted a graduate degree concurrently with their basic professional qualification.

Requests for additional information about any of these programs should be submitted to the directors of specific programs. A listing of these programs can be obtained from the APTA and is also printed periodically in *Physical Therapy,* which is the official publication of the APTA.

Final entry into the profession is obtained on successful completion of the requirements for state licensure or registration. The primary criterion for licensure in most states is the successful completion of an examination that evaluates the applicant's knowledge in the categories of basic science, clinical science, and physical therapy procedures. If an individual has been licensed or registered in one state it may be possible through the process of endorsement to become licensed or registered in another state without reexamination.

SUPPORTIVE PERSONNEL

The APTA has developed two categories of supportive personnel to assist the physical therapist; these are the physical therapist assistant and the physical therapy aide.

The assistant's education consists of a two-year educational program in an approved and accredited community, technical, or junior college. The program contains preprofessional and professional course work, some of which may be transferable for credit toward a degree in physical therapy. However, the assistant curriculum is not considered the most appropriate preparatory work for a baccalaureate program. Completion of the program terminates with the granting of an associate degree, but it is possible for the assistant eventually to become enrolled in a baccalaureate program.

The assistant is employed to perform specific administrative and patient care activities under the supervision of the physical therapist. Primary evaluation procedures, preparation of entire treatment programs, or total departmental administration are not responsibilities assigned to the assistant. The assistant may be required to become licensed, registered, or certified in order to meet state requirements. The APTA has a membership category for assistants, and they have been granted many rights and privileges within the APTA.

The physical therapy aide possesses a high school diploma and receives on-the-job training within the physical therapy department through in-service education programs under the supervision of a qualified physical therapist. The aide functions under the direct supervision of the therapist and is given responsibilities in equipment care and maintenance, supply requisition, housekeeping duties, department and patient preparation for treatment, and minor departmental administrative activities. Aides do not receive any formal recognition by the APTA on completion of the training program and cannot become APTA members.

PERSONAL QUALITIES

Since physical therapists work directly with people to perform the majority of their professional activities, those considering the profession as a career should have an inherent desire to assist others. They should be aware of and sensitive to the physical, psychological, social, cultural, and personal needs of those with whom they work. The most effective therapists are people who are able to adjust and adapt to various patient personalities or disabilities while maintaining their own personal emotional stability. The therapist will be required to exhibit appropriate judgment, decision-making skills, common sense, and leadership in many routine and emergency situations. Reliability, dependability, conscientiousness, internal motivation, initiative, and creativity are attributes that enhance the physical therapist's ability to work effectively. (See Fig. 28.)

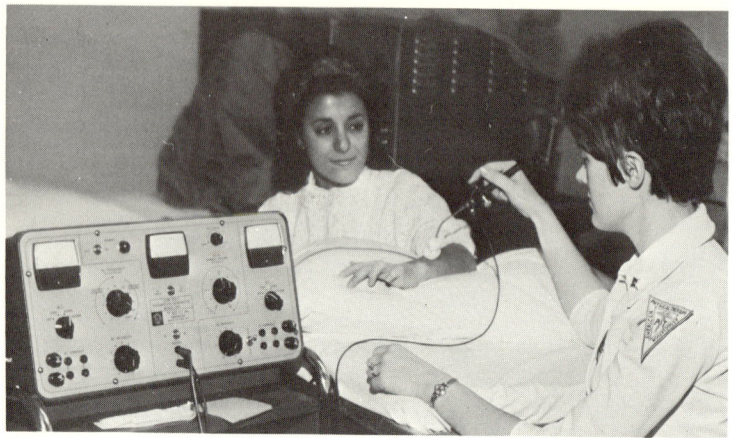

Fig. 28. The physical therapist uses electrical stimulation both for evaluation and muscle reeducation.

Age, sex, or stature are not limiting factors in the performance of professional activities, provided the individual maintains normal standards of physical health. These include strength, endurance, and motor skills appropriate to the performance of sustained vigorous work.

EMPLOYMENT OPPORTUNITIES

Physical therapists are employed in various types of facilities and environments, and the profession is an integral component of the health care delivery system. Most therapists are salaried employees of a hospital, but other employment opportunities include work in clinics, community agencies (for example, the Arthritis Foundation, Easter Seal Societies for Crippled Children and Adults, National Elks Foundation), local and state public health programs, physicians' offices, and federal and state agencies and institutions (including the armed services). The salary range for these positions is usually between $9,000 and $11,000 annually for the recent graduate who requires supervision from an experienced therapist. The experienced staff therapist may earn from $11,000 to $13,000 annually, while a supervising therapist may earn from $13,000 to $16,000, and a departmental director may earn from $15,000 to $20,000. These ranges vary according to local economics, the demand for therapists, and similar factors.

Some experienced therapists serve as consultants to nursing homes, rural hospitals, and other types of facilities that offer a limited range of services. Their role may be to provide guidance in developing physical therapy in the facility through the education and training of personnel, or they may provide direct patient care.

It is also possible for the physical therapist to be an independent practitioner and treat clients in an office, in the client's home, or in a skilled nursing facility through the use of a physician's referral. Increased income for the self-employed therapist as compared to that of the salaried therapist is one advantage of this type of practice.

A limited number of therapists are active in sports medicine and serve as athletic trainers for high school, college, or university and professional sports activities.

Physical therapists with graduate degrees and extensive clinical experience are frequently employed as educators on the physical therapy faculties of the existing professional and physical therapist assistant programs. The need for teachers has increased recently due to the development of additional programs and an increased student enrollment within many of the existing programs.

Part-time employment is available to the physical therapist, since there is usually a greater demand for the service than can be provided by the available number of full-time therapists. Many therapists who are inactive have been encouraged to return to the profession to help fulfill the need for additional personnel and have been provided with "refresher courses" to update their skills and previous knowledge.

In 1974 there were approximately 15,000 members of the APTA and 20,000 qualified physical therapists in the United States. The annual attrition rate due to retirement and other factors is about 20%, while the annual number of physical therapy graduates of all programs is approximately 1,900. It has been estimated that a 30% increase in the total number of employed therapists would be required to provide adequate delivery of physical therapy services in the United States.

The role of the physical therapist continues to expand because of the influence of recent revisions in federal health care legislation, the impact of the independent practitioner, and the need to provide the services requested by the consumers of health care services. Physical therapists are now expected to perform more sophisticated evaluative procedures, to use an interdisciplinary approach to improve total patient care, and to assume increased responsibilities of patient treatment, program planning, and implementation.

PROFESSIONAL CONTRIBUTIONS TO HEALTH CARE

The physical therapist as a member of the health care delivery group must actively participate in the direct and indirect treatment of a wide variety of patient problems. Specific treatment skills include the use of therapeutic exercise, massage, communication, and the use of physical agents (heat, cold, water, electricity, and sound). (See Fig. 29.) These skills are used to assist the person with musculoskeletal (fractures, muscular strains, amputations, arthritis, etc.), neurological (strokes, paralysis, spinal cord injuries, etc.), and cardiopulmonary (emphysema, hypertension, asthma, etc.) problems as well as many other specific physical limitations. Additional skills required are those involved in the

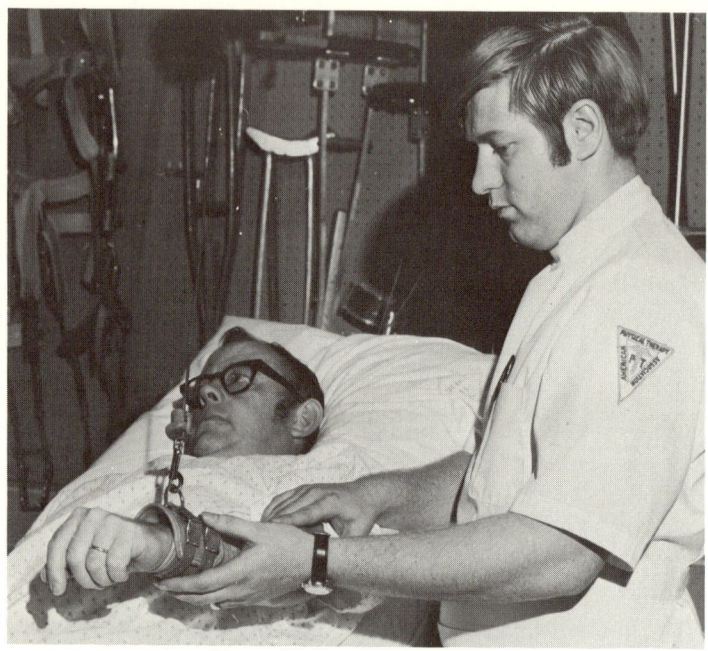

Fig. 29. Developing strength, coordination, and endurance of major muscle groups is part of rehabilitation.

evaluation of patient problems, program development and implementation, and general administrative activities.

Therapists are also involved with patient and staff conferences, special clinics, and teaching activities. They have a responsibility to inform other members of the health care team of their professional knowledge of the patient and must be able to correlate the information received from other health professionals to their management of patients. Administratively, the therapist is required to complete various types of patient records, including status notes, attendance data, scheduling and census records, treatment procedures performed, and patient data for billing purposes.

The following hypothetical case study has been designed to illustrate some of the responsibilities and activities in which the physical therapist engages while providing direct patient care.

>J. D., a 20-year-old man, was admitted to the hospital following a motorcycle accident that caused irreparable damage to his spinal cord. This produced loss of motor and sensory function to the muscles, organs, and tissues below the level of his waist.
>
>Two weeks after admission the physical therapist received a physician referral that requested an evaluation of J. D. and the development of a program to improve his functional independence.

Initial physical therapy treatments were performed in J. D.'s room and were designed to promote range of motion of the joints in his legs and hips and to strengthen the muscles of his arms and shoulders. Proper bed positioning and a schedule for turning were instituted with assistance from the nursing service to avoid muscular contractures and skin breakdown.

When he was able to be moved from his room, J. D. was treated in the rehabilitation unit of the physical therapy department. Arm strengthening activities were continued, while activities to develop sitting balance and wheelchair mobility were initiated. He was taught to protect his skin below the level of the spinal cord lesion from injury and pressure to avoid skin breakdown.

J. D. was eventually fitted with temporary leg splints to provide knee stability so he could attempt standing and minimal ambulation exercises in the parallel bars. He also received additional instructions in wheelchair mobility skills that improved his independence.

The occupational therapist instructed J. D. in adapted techniques of dressing and personal hygiene. He was also evaluated for his manual dexterity and manipulative skills in preparation for educational and vocational counseling.

Through the combined efforts of the occupational therapist, physical therapist, and driving instructor, J. D. was taught how to transfer from his wheelchair into the car, place his wheelchair in the car, and drive with special hand controls to operate the brake and accelerator.

He became interested in wheelchair athletics and participated in basketball, track and field events, Ping Pong, archery, and swimming. He not only gained pleasure from these recreational activities but also improved his wheelchair skills, increased his endurance for physical activity, and gained a new self-confidence in his ability to interact with others.

At the time J. D. was discharged from the hospital, he was independent in all normal activities of feeding, dressing, personal hygiene, wheelchair mobility, and transfers. He was well aware of his physical abilities and was preparing to return to college.

SUMMARY

The primary activities of the physical therapist are those associated with direct patient care of persons of all ages (infants to the elderly). The basic components of patient care for which the therapist is responsible are evaluation or assessment of the patient's functional capacities, development of objectives of treatment, program planning based on the predetermined objectives, implementation of the treatment program, and periodic reevaluation of the patient's functional capacities. The physical therapist must be able to work with the patient and the family to plan a program that will restore the patient to the highest possible level of independent functioning within the limits imposed by the patient's disability, whether it is the result of disease, trauma, or congenital factors. In addition to specific physical needs, concern is also given to the patient's social, economic, vocational, educational, and recreational needs.

The physical therapist works in cooperation with other health professionals, including nurses, occupational therapists, social workers, respiratory technologists, medical dietitians, and speech therapists. Guidance in the development of treatment programs is obtained from a licensed physician or dentist through written referrals or prescriptions and personal consultations.

SUGGESTED READINGS

American Medical Association Council on Medical Education: Allied medical education directory, Chicago, 1974, American Medical Association.

Handbook for physical therapy teachers, Washington, D.C., 1967, American Physical Therapy Association.

Krumhansl, B.: Opportunities in physical therapy, Louisville, Ky., 1974, Vocational Guidance Manuals, Inc.

Physical Therapy, Journal of the American Physical Therapy Association.

PROFESSIONAL ORGANIZATION WHERE FURTHER INFORMATION CAN BE OBTAINED

American Physical Therapy Association
1156 15th Street, N.W.
Washington, D.C. 20005

Chapter 18

Physician's assistant

Monica V. Brown

The physician's assistant is one of the newest and most challenging careers among the allied health professions. The term "physician's assistant" is generic. There have been assistants to the physician since the time of Hippocrates in the fifth century B.C. However, the concept of the physician's assistant as a distinctive profession was first introduced in 1966 at Duke University in Durham, North Carolina. The first four students, all of whom were former military corpsmen, were chosen because of their education and experience during military service in caring for people with health problems. They represented an unused manpower resource in the civilian health care field. In 1969 the first MEDEX* program, designed to educate former military corpsmen for civilian health service, was initiated by the University of Washington and funded by the federal government.

The first graduates of these programs were seen as supportive personnel working with physicians wherever they went, be it the hospital, operating room, private office, clinic, or patients' homes. Physician's assistants now work in all of these areas. Most are employed directly by private physicians. Some, however, are employed by hospitals, nursing homes, extended care facilities, and health clinics, where they work under the supervision of physicians. They administer care to patients in these facilities. The assistant role is a dependent one, but the implications are very broad since physicians may delegate to the assistant all of the tasks they feel can be performed by that person. This means that physician's assistants often carry out many functions that were formerly the exclusive province of the physician.

In 1970 the National Academy of Sciences developed three categories of physician's assistants. Type A assistants are capable of performing physical examinations, taking histories, and organizing data to help physicians diagnose problems. They are also capable of assisting

---

*MEDEX is an acronym for *médecin extension,* a French term indicating the extension of the physician's care. Following the return from Vietnam of hundreds of medical corpsmen with excellent skills in a variety of emergency and general medical techniques, the MEDEX program was designed as a supplement to Armed Services Medical Corps training and field experience to produce primary care physician's assistants.

in the performance of various diagnostic and therapeutic procedures as well as in coordinating total patient care. The type A assistant is a medical generalist distinguished by the ability to exercise a degree of independent judgment. Assistants to primary care physicians are type A. Type B assistants, while not equipped with knowledge and skills relative to the whole range of medical care, are persons who possess exceptional skill in one clinical specialty or, more commonly, in certain procedures within such a specialty. Examples of the type B assistant are surgical assistants, ophthalmic assistants, and orthopedic assistants. Type C assistants perform many tasks of a general nature, but they do not possess the medical knowledge necessary to interpret findings.

Most educational and training programs for physician's assistants fall into the type A and B categories, with the majority being type A assistants who work in primary, preventive, and emergency medicine alongside family practitioners, pediatricians, and internists.

In December of 1970 the American Medical Association defined the physician's assistant as "a skilled person qualified by academic and practical on-the-job training to provide patient services under the supervision and direction of a licensed physician, who is responsible for the performance of the assistant." Standards for the education of physician's assistants were then established by the American Medical Association Council on Medical Education, which acts in collaboration with the various medical specialty boards to accredit programs for physician's assistants. Three types of programs are presently being accredited: assistant to the primary care physician, urologic physician's assistant, and surgeon's assistant.

In the ten years that have passed since the first program was introduced, more than eighty physician's assistant programs have been developed. Fifty-six of these educate assistants to primary care physicians. In 1974 the class capacity of forty-three AMA-approved programs was 1,300 annually. As of July, 1975, forty-nine programs had been approved by the AMA. Several hundred graduates are already working, and job opportunities are plentiful. The greatest needs are in the area of primary, preventive, and emergency care. In 1974, patients of physicians employing assistants in their practices were surveyed to determine their attitude toward these new personnel. Of those who responded, 89% were pleased with the physician's assistant. In one decade, the physician's assistant has become a recognized allied health professional.

EDUCATION

Variety is the keynote in physician's assistant programs. The courses of instruction vary in length from one to four years, with two-year programs the most common. A high school diploma or the equivalent is required by all programs, and direct experience in patient care is important. Satisfactory SAT and ACT scores are additional factors considered. A number of schools require college credits. As the profession becomes a more familiar part of the health care system, increasing numbers of students are seeking careers as physician's assistants and more programs are welcoming the high school graduate who meets the necessary prerequisites for entrance into the program. Credentials awarded on completion of the program range from certificates to associate and baccalaureate degrees. The number of students accepted into each class varies between ten and fifty; the average class size is fifteen. The curriculum includes didactic instruction and clinical practicums in anatomy, pediatrics, family medicine, and general procedures including physical examinations and patient histories.

Graduates of physician's assistant programs have the opportunity to move from the role of generalist to that of specialist. Likewise, those who have graduated from specialty assistant programs may continue their education into the general medical areas.

CREDENTIALS

In December of 1973 the National Board of Medical Examiners administered the first tests for national certification of primary care physician's assistants. Graduates of AMA-approved programs as well as those who have gained their education and training outside the formal route may now apply for and take the national certification examinations. Graduates are being recognized in an increasing number of states as those able to practice as physician's assistants under the jurisdiction of a licensed physician within those states. In 1974 the National Commission on Certification of Physician's Assistants was established. This is the body now responsible for certifying physician's assistants. The certifying examination given annually includes both written and performance components.

More than forty states now have legislation regarding physician's assistants. In other states the matter is under consideration, and increasing numbers of states recognize those who have passed the examination of the National Commission on Certification of Physician's Assistants.

SUMMARY

Physician's assistants are competent, understanding professionals who are educated and trained to assist the physician by performing diagnostic and therapeutic procedures and coordinating the role of other more technical assistants.

There will certainly be some modifications in this allied health profession, which has raced from birth to maturity in ten short years, but the physician's assistant is now an accepted member of the health team. According to present projections, these professionals will become increasingly useful in the delivery of health care.

REFERENCES

Kacen, A.: Examining job prospects and training for physician's assistants, Occupational Outlook Quarterly **18:**17, 1974.

Nelson, E. C., Jacobs, A. R., and Johnson, K. G.: Patients' acceptance of physician's assistants, Journal of the American Medical Association **228:** 63, 1974.

SUGGESTED READINGS

Sadler, A. M., Jr., Sadler, B. L., and Bliss, A. A.: The physician's assistant today and tomorrow, New Haven, Conn., 1972, Yale University Press.

PROFESSIONAL ORGANIZATIONS WHERE FURTHER INFORMATION CAN BE OBTAINED

American Academy of Physician's Assistants and Association of Physician's Assistant Programs
2120 L Street, N.W.
Washington, D.C. 20037

American Medical Association
535 North Dearborn Street
Chicago, Illinois 60610

National Commission on Certification of Physician's Assistants
338 H Peachtree Road, N.E.
Atlanta, Georgia 30326

Chapter 19
Podiatry
William F. Munsey

Podiatry is the health science profession dealing with the examination, diagnosis, treatment, prevention, and care of conditions and functions of the human foot. This care is realized through the utilization of medical, surgical, mechanical, or physical means.

HISTORY OF THE PROFESSION

The profession of podiatric medicine is one of the oldest medical arts. Perhaps the earliest podiatric care began with cavemen who wrapped their feet with animal skins as protection from the elements and rough ground. There is also evidence of rudimentary foot care in ancient times, especially in ancient Egypt. The first recorded references to foot problems were made by the Greeks in the fourth century B.C. The modern specialty of podiatric medicine, however, can trace its beginnings to medieval times when the guilds or barber-surgeons— itinerant practitioners of primitive surgery, dentistry, and other pseudoscientific procedures—attempted to work their "skills" for beautification as well as healing.

Gradually podiatric medicine underwent its metamorphosis, and today it is a profession that forms a separate, distinct, and complementary division of the healing arts.

The term "chiropodist" was introduced in England in 1774. It was coined by David Low, who had authored a book entitled *Chiropodologia*. The word originates from the Latin *chirugen*, or surgeon, and *pod*, or foot; thus a chiropodist was a surgeon of the foot. In 1917 the profession adopted the term "podiatrist," and both chiropody and podiatry were used interchangeably until World War II. Today, podiatry is the accepted term.

Among the earliest foot specialists in the United States were Julius Davidson, who opened an office in Philadelphia in 1841, and Dr. Nehemiah Kenison, who started in Boston in 1846 and soon had branch offices in many eastern cities.

At the time of the Civil War, Dr. Isacher Zacharie wrote the first text on chiropody published in the United States. As President Lincoln's personal chiropodist, Dr. Zacharie served on several occasions as an emissary for the President, who is reputed to have recommended him for the commission "Chiropodist-General of the United States Army."

The maturation of the profession began in earnest in 1911 with the establishment of the first school of podiatry in New York City. One year later the National Association of Chiropodists was established. In 1912 the Illinois College of Chiropody and Orthopedics began offering a course in surgical chiropody and mechanical foot orthopedics. In 1916 the Ohio College of Chiropody began training foot specialists.

The national professional organization is now called the American Podiatry Association (APA). There are now six colleges of podiatric medicine in the United States accredited by the Council on Podiatry Education of the APA and recognized by the United States Office of Education and the National Commission on Accrediting. The newest college began accepting students in the fall of 1975.

CAREERS IN PODIATRY

Of the approximately 8,500 podiatrists in the United States, nearly 85% are engaged in private practice. Although podiatrists have traditionally been engaged in solo practice, the trend is now changing and group practices are more common.

The average podiatrist practices the full scope of his profession, ranging from the routine care of chronic problems such as corns, calluses, warts, ingrown toenails, and injuries, to extended foot surgery. (See Fig. 30.)

In addition to private practice, podiatrists serve on the staffs of

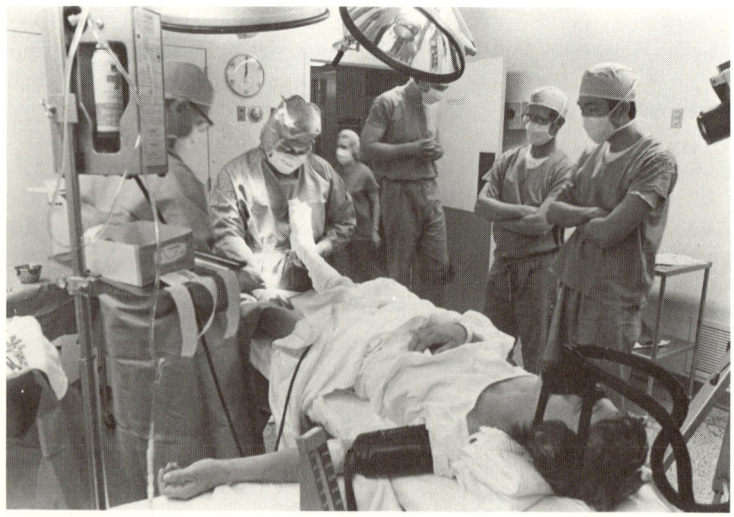

Fig. 30. The podiatrist inspects dressings following completion of foot surgery. (Courtesy American Podiatry Association, Washington, D.C.)

nursing homes, hospitals, and extended care facilities accredited by the Joint Commission on Accreditation of Hospitals and Nursing Homes and the American Osteopathic Association. Podiatrists also serve on the faculties of the colleges of podiatric medicine, medical schools and nursing schools, in the Armed Forces, and in municipal health departments.

Podiatrists are often the first to diagnose systemic diseases, including arthritis, heart disease, kidney ailments, and arteriosclerosis. Whenever such symptoms are detected, the foot specialist consults with the patient's medical doctor concerning continuing treatment.

PERSONAL QUALITIES

Podiatry offers a rewarding career for both men and women who sincerely care for people and wish to devote their lives to the relief of human suffering. It is also a unique profession in that the majority of patients seen daily leave the office with immediate relief from the symptoms with which they entered.

It is also an uncrowded profession, with approximately 3.5 podiatrists for every 100,000 population, a figure that falls far short of providing services to the millions of people who have some type of foot disorder.

Recent surveys indicate that most podiatrists practice by appointment, working forty-eight to fifty weeks per year. The average net income after three years of practice is in excess of $30,000 annually.

EDUCATIONAL PREPARATION

Published minimum standards for admission to a college of podiatric medicine are sixty semester hours or ninety quarter hours of accredited undergraduate study. More than 85% of the students in professional training, however, have baccalaureate degrees at the time of entrance. The remainder of the successful candidates have three or more years of accredited college work.

Each applicant's preprofessional college credits must include a one-year course or the equivalent in each of the following subjects: English, general chemistry, and general biology or zoology, and one-half year of organic chemistry and physics. While these standards are nearly universal at all colleges of podiatric medicine, it would be well to inquire at a specific college for complete requirements. In addition, a satisfactory score on the Colleges of Podiatry Admission Test (CPAT) is a preadmission requirement.

The professional training, a four-year course, is very similar to that of a medical college. Students in their junior and senior years receive extensive clinical training. Graduates are awarded the degree of Doctor of Podiatric Medicine and may apply for residency programs that are one, two, or three years in length. As a general rule, the first-year residency is a general program, and the two- and three-year programs specialize in foot surgery. These programs are conducted at the colleges of podiatric medicine and in Joint Commission–accredited hospitals, as well as in those accredited by the American Osteopathic Association.

Graduates are required to take a state board examination in order to practice in a particular state. The profession also has a National Podiatry Board examination that is accepted in many states.

SUPPORTING PERSONNEL

Podiatry assistants play an important role, and there are now two formal educational programs. Jefferson College in Kentucky offers a two-year program leading to an associate in arts degree. The Pennsylvania College of Podiatric Medicine in Philadelphia conducts the other two-year program.

SUMMARY

Podiatry is a relatively new profession that has rapidly earned the acceptance of the general public and the other health professions. Current podiatry education is comparable to training offered in other schools for health professionals, and the field today offers unique opportunities for its practitioners, including women and members of all ethnic groups.

REFERENCES

Approved podiatric residency programs 1974-75, Washington, D.C., 1974, Council on Podiatry Education, American Podiatry Association.

Characteristics of patients treated by podiatrists, D.H.E.W. Publication No. (HRA) 751809, Rockville, Md., 1974, United States Department of Health, Education, and Welfare, Public Health Service, Health Resources Administration, National Center for Health Statistics.

Podiatry manpower: characteristics of clinical practice, United States, 1970, Rockville, Md., 1973, United States Department of Health, Education and Welfare, Public Health Service, Health Resources Administration.

SUGGESTED READINGS

Feinberg, H.: Podiatric medicine: professional profile, Journal of the American Optometric Association **41:**454, 1970.

PROFESSIONAL ORGANIZATION WHERE FURTHER INFORMATION CAN BE OBTAINED

The American Podiatry Association
20 Chevy Chase Circle, N.W.
Washington, D.C. 20015

Chapter 20

Radiologic technology

J. Robert Bullock and Philip W. Ballinger

Almost every patient admitted to a hospital requires some type of X-ray examination. This service may vary from a routine chest film to an elaborate study of one of the body systems that involves tremendously complicated and expensive equipment. Whether the examination is simple or complex, the final results represent the combined efforts of the radiologist (a physician whose specialty is the use of X-rays and other radiation in diagnosis and treatment) and a radiologic technologist.

DEVELOPMENT OF THE PROFESSION

Few events have had as great an impact on the medical world as the discovery of X-rays in 1895. Physicians immediately realized the potential of this new energy that would allow them to see inside the patient. Therefore those with the necessary mechanical and technical abilities worked with physicists and other scientists, and within a year significant X-ray studies were being performed on patients.

The first radiographs (X-ray photographs) resulted from the combined efforts of physicians and physicists. At this stage the physicists operated crude X-ray generating equipment while the physician positioned the patient and evaluated the image on the finished glass plate. Soon X-ray equipment was being manufactured commercially, and more refined equipment became available.

As the practices of radiologists began to expand, they developed an increasing need for competent people who could assume responsibility for much of the technical work involved in performing radiographic studies, allowing the radiologist to focus his efforts on the interpretation of films and other professional duties that must be performed by a physician.

While physicians were developing the field of radiology as a medical specialty, X-ray technicians were being trained in the technical aspects of obtaining a radiograph. The introduction of radioactivity and the increased sophistication of therapeutic and diagnositc procedures required expanded educational programs. Through more demanding educational requirements and added responsibilities, these technical people were accumulating the knowledge and skills that distinguish today's radiologic technologists.

Since its inception, the field of radiology has developed with remarkable rapidity. This progress has resulted from the development of new techniques by clinicians, mechanical and electronic contributions by the X-ray industry, and the continuing development and refinement of radiopaque contrast materials by the pharmaceutical industry.

The radiologist of the 1920s and 1930s studied images on a fluoroscopic screen—images so dim they could be seen only in a room that was totally dark. By the late 1950s, image intensifiers capable of increasing the brightness of the fluoroscopic image 6,000 times had become available. This image intensifier now permits the use of television, motion picture cameras, and videotape to transmit or record studies of organs where motion is involved. This system can demonstrate the valves and blood vessels of the heart with great clarity, and it can also be used to great advantage for the more traditional studies of the gastrointestinal tract.

In certain respects the radiologic technologist is a representative of, as well as an assistant to, the radiologist. Radiologic examinations may be divided into two general categories: those performed by a radiologist because medical judgments are involved in the performance of the study and those in which the technologist produces radiographs that are later interpreted by a radiologist. In the latter case the patient will frequently be seen only by the technologist. This situation is particularly common in rural or small community hospitals where a radiologist may consult only on a part-time basis. Under these circumstances technologists must function with greater independence, judgment, and responsibility because they are often the only members of the health care team with any expertise in the field.

DIAGNOSTIC RADIOLOGY

When a patient is directed to the radiology department for a diagnostic study, the patient is greeted by the technologist, who prepares him for the examination. Preparation usually includes an explanation of the procedure to allay the patient's anxiety and elicit cooperation.

In order to obtain a radiograph, technologists must position the patient precisely to project the desired anatomical structures onto the film. To accomplish this they must relate external body landmarks to internal structures. (See Fig. 31.) The technologist must evaluate the patient's weight, age, and physical condition in order to select the proper X-ray exposure values. The film will then be exposed and sent to the darkroom to be processed by personnel under the technologist's supervision. Finished films are prepared for the radiologist's interpretation and are ultimately filed.

Radiologic technologists are responsible for patients during their stay in the radiology department, and some patients require considerable supportive care. In addition to working directly with patients, technologists must supervise the maintenance of equipment to ensure

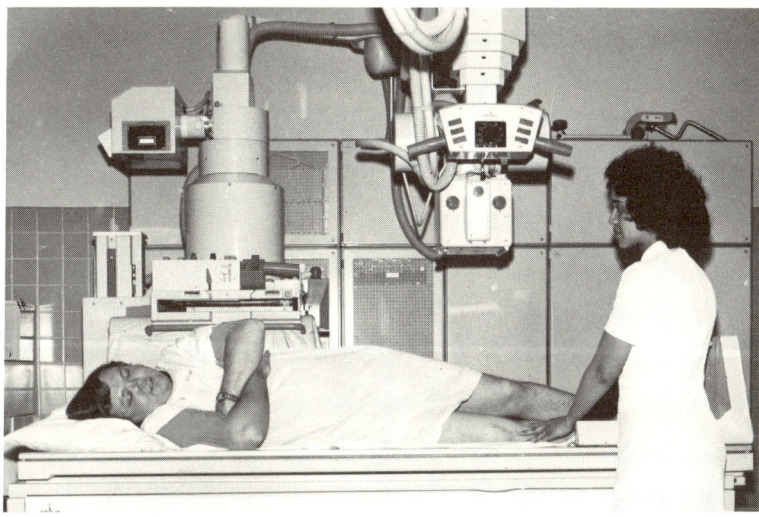

Fig. 31. Precise positioning of the patient is essential to project the desired anatomical structure on the radiograph or X-ray film.

dependable function, test new products, and maintain an appropriate inventory of expendable supplies. In some institutions they may be called on to participate in developing new techniques to assist in research programs.

Radiologic technology can be thought of as an art, and in this respect it can be highly rewarding. A well-composed and properly exposed radiograph that clearly reveals the anatomy in question can appropriately be compared to an example of any of the graphic arts. In addition, technologists have the satisfaction of knowing that the information revealed will be essential to the patient's care and treatment. Personal satisfaction is also derived from performing difficult radiographic studies without causing additional discomfort to a patient who is already in pain. Radiographic examinations may range from relatively routine films to those urgently required in the emergency room or during surgery. In some cases, portable radiographic equipment is taken to the patient whose condition does not allow him to be moved to the radiology department.

The following case study illustrates the radiologic technologist's role in the care of one patient.

> Mrs. H. fell down the front steps of her home and was taken to the hospital emergency room, where she was examined by her physician. He detected a probable hip injury and directed a request for a hip study to the radiology department. Mrs. H. was taken to an X-ray room and carefully moved onto the radiographic table.

The technologist placed film in a tray under the radiographic table and moved the X-ray tube above the patient, centering it over her injured hip. The technologist was careful not to cause her further injury. After the initial exposure was made, the technologist moved the equipment so that a second projection could be made without moving the patient and risking additional pain and injury. Special devices were required to hold the second film at the patient's side, with the X-ray tube placed at right angles to the hip joint. Care was taken to move only the uninjured leg so that the injured area remained stationary. After the films were processed, the physician interpreted them and confirmed that Mrs. H.'s hip was fractured. Her physician informed her of the diagnosis; she was admitted to the orthopedic service and scheduled for surgery.

Immediately before the surgical repair of Mrs. H.'s hip was begun, the radiologic technologist joined the other members of the surgical team in the operating room to take preliminary films. The information provided by these radiographs permitted the surgeon to correctly adjust the injured hip and initiate surgery. When the incision revealed bony structure, the surgeon placed a guide wire into the fractured hip and the technologist took additional films. When the films indicated that the wire was satisfactorily located and did not require additional manipulation, the surgeon attached the repair device to the fractured hip by sliding it over the guide wire. After the permanent pin or plate was installed, the guide wire was removed and another series of radiographs were taken. When the films showed satisfactory placement, the surgeon closed the incision. Mrs. H was kept under close observation immediately following surgery and subsequent films were taken to monitor her recovery.

THERAPEUTIC RADIOLOGY

The therapeutic application of X-rays parallels the development of diagnostic radiology. The first therapeutic use of X-rays was reported in 1896. Since that time there has been an increased understanding of radiobiology and continuous development of higher energy generators and radioactive treatment sources with different and more effective modalities.

Technologists in radiotherapy work under the direction of a radiologist. They assist in checking calculations involving the treatment and position the patient so that the radiation source and the area to be irradiated are in proper alignment. They regulate the controls of the radiation source to deliver the exact amount of radiation to be administered and observe the patient continually during the treatment period either through a television monitoring system or directly through lead glass windows. Technologists also assist the physician in regular examinations of patients to chart their progress. Assisting the radiologist in planning treatment programs is an interesting and challenging part of their activities. Many technologists prefer to work in therapeutic radiology because the longer association with a patient provides opportunities for technologists to see the results of their contributions to patient care.

NUCLEAR MEDICINE

Nuclear medicine is a product of the atomic age. In this medical specialty, radionuclides (radioactive pharmaceuticals) are administered to the patient, whose body is then scanned with a device that detects radiation emitted from organs or areas where the nuclide may have collected. An imaging device records the patterns of radioactivity on a film that the physician can use to diagnose tumors or other disease entities. In addition, tests of various biochemical and physiological functions are performed. Because the nuclides that are used are active for only a limited time, patients commonly experience no ill aftereffects.

Nuclear medicine technologists may prepare the selected nuclide and administer it to a patient under the direction of a physician. They also operate the imaging device and produce the resultant scan film. People with a special interest in physics who enjoy precise laboratory work and complex instrumentation find this aspect of radiology especially attractive.

EDUCATIONAL PREPARATION

The American Association of Radiological Technicians, the first professional organization for allied health personnel in radiology, was founded in 1920. This organization whose official title is now the American Society of Radiologic Technologists (ASRT), has worked continuously to develop and improve curriculums in schools of radiologic technology. The American Registry of Radiologic Technologists (ARRT), sponsored by the American College of Radiology and the ASRT, examines and certifies graduate technologists. Successful candidates earn the title of registered technologist and use the abbreviation R.T. following their names. As the field of radiology continued to expand, the ARRT recognized the need for additional education and certification for radiation therapy and nuclear medicine technologists.

Today there are well over 1,000 AMA-approved programs in diagnostic radiography, and approximately 100 each in the specialties of radiation therapy and nuclear medicine technology in the United States. While there is an increasing trend toward two-year associate degree and four-year baccalaureate programs, the majority of schools are hospital-based certificate programs. The objective of most baccalaureate programs is to produce technically competent professionals with the additional preparation needed to assume administrative or teaching positions. All AMA-approved programs include didactic instruction in conjunction with extensive clinical instruction. The total length of an educational program must be at least twenty-four months, and graduates of all AMA-approved programs are eligible to apply for certification by the ARRT. To qualify for admission to a diagnostic radiologic technology program, one must be a high school graduate with preparation in mathematics and science.

Schools following the curriculum suggested by the ASRT offer courses in the following areas:

Radiation protection
X-ray physics
Anatomy and physiology
Principles of radiographic exposure
Darkroom chemistry
Principles of radiation therapy
Principles of nuclear medicine
Orientation to the operating room
Nursing procedures
Standard and special radiographic positioning
Special radiographic procedures
Ethics

Candidates for admission to programs that offer instruction in radiation therapy technology may be either graduates of approved schools of radiologic technology or registered nurses who have successfully completed a course in radiation physics. Students who are accepted into these programs spend a minimum of twelve months to become eligible to take a registry examination in radiation therapy technology. Some radiation therapy programs offer two years of concentrated studies. Applicants must be high school graduates. Those who achieve satisfactory scores on the registry examination become registered radiation therapy technologists.

Accredited schools of nuclear medicine technology consider candidates who are registered medical laboratory technologists, registered radiologic technologists, registered nurses, or individuals with a baccalaureate degree from an accredited college with a major in the biological or physical sciences. On completion of the one-year program of combined instruction and clinical experience, graduates are eligible to apply for the registry examination in nuclear medicine technology.

Technologists who have earned certification following a minimum of twenty-four months of education but who do not have professional work experience will find that starting salaries vary according to geographical area, size of the community, and availability of registered technologists. Radiologic technologists' salaries in general are comparable to those offered to similarly educated allied health professionals.

SUMMARY

Approved schools graduate approximately 7,000 students each year, but far greater numbers are needed to supply technologists for the more than 7,000 hospitals, 5,000 clinics, and several thousand laboratories in private offices. Opportunities exist in rural areas as well as in urban centers.

Those considering careers in radiologic technology must have compassion for the sick and injured. Emotional maturity is essential if the technologist is to work effectively in the hospital environment.

REFERENCE

Grigg, E. R. N.: The trail of the invisible light, Springfield, Ill., 1965, Charles C Thomas, Publisher.

SUGGESTED READINGS

Donizetti, P.: Shadow and substance, New York, 1967, Pergamon Press.

Grigg, E. R. N.: The new history of radiology, Radiologic Technology **36:**229, 1965.

Horizons unlimited, ed. 8, Chicago, 1970, American Medical Association.

Roth, C. J., and Weimer, L.: Hospital health services, New York, 1964, Henry Z. Walck, Inc.

The challenge—radiologic technology. The future—yours, New York, 1968, E. R. Squibb & Sons, Inc.

X-rays and you, Rochester, N.Y. 1965, Eastman Kodak Co.

PROFESSIONAL ORGANIZATIONS WHERE FURTHER INFORMATION CAN BE OBTAINED

American Society of Radiologic Technologists
Suite 836
500 North Michigan Avenue
Chicago, Illinois 60611

American Registry of Radiologic Technologists
2600 Wayzata Boulevard
Minneapolis, Minnesota 55405

Chapter 21

Respiratory therapy

O. Theodore Haaland

Respiratory therapy involves assistance in the diagnosis and care of heart and lung system disorders in patients of all age groups in hospitals as well as at patients' homes. Most respiratory therapy currently is practiced in the country's general, acute care hospitals and consists fundamentally of the administration of oxygen and oxygen mixtures by various breathing devices, application of mechanical ventilators of several types to assist or control breathing patterns, and provision of breathable fogs to help maintain open lung passages.

Many variations of these techniques exist, and adjunctive activities extend the respiratory therapist's skills much beyond this scope. Additional major tasks include diagnostic testing of breathing function, physical manipulation to enhance lung cleansing, exercise programs designed to improve physical abilities, participation in cardiopulmonary resuscitation, and monitoring of the heart and lung function of critically ill patients. Some common respiratory therapy activities are discussed in detail later in this chapter.

SCIENTIFIC HISTORY

Concern with the mystery of "breath as life" is apparent early in human history, but the development of a cadre of health professionals dedicated to the amelioration of respiratory ills is a quite recent occurrence. The tale of the biblical prophet Elijah's apparent use of mouth-to-mouth resuscitation is fairly well known, as are the experiments of Aristotle in the fourth century B.c in which small animals were observed to die when placed in airtight boxes. The fifteenth-century anatomist Andreas Vesalius maintained heart pulsations and life in an animal by blowing into a hollow reed he inserted in its trachea. The experimental efforts of the seventeenth-century English chemists, notably Robert Boyle and Robert Hooke, greatly enhanced scientific interest in mammalian respiration and expanded knowledge of the physical nature and activity of gases. Toward the latter part of the eighteenth century, just prior to the American Revolution, "dephlogisticated air"* (named in accordance with the erroneous hypotheses

---

*George Ernst Stahl, professor of physiology at Halle, Germany, propounded an erroneous theory in which a substance called phlogiston was thought to be given off during combustion. Stahl's hypothesis bedeviled chemistry for decades, and Priestly never forsook his adherence to it, having failed to draw correct conclusions from his numerous gas experiments.

then current) was produced in the laboratory of Joseph Priestley as well as by the Swedish chemist Scheele. Priestley's notes regarding experiments with this gas—shortly to be named oxygen by the brilliant Frenchman Antoine Lavoisier—are piquant:

> My reader will not wonder that, having ascertained the superior goodness of dephlogisticated air by mice living in it, and the other tests mentioned above, I should have the curiosity to taste it myself.... I have gratified that curiosity by breathing it, drawing it through a glass syphon, and by this means I reduced a large jar full of it to the standard of common air, but I fancied that my breath felt peculiarly light and easy for some time afterwards. Who can tell but that in time this pure air may become a fashionable article in luxury. Hitherto, only two mice and myself have had the privilege of breathing it.*

The discovery of oxygen and other medical gases set the stage for the first serious (and some not-so-serious) attempts at providing a beneficient artificial atmosphere for human inhalation. Thomas Beddoes, an English physician, held that a wide variety of disorders could be relieved by the breathing of manufactured airs of varying gas content, and in 1798 he established the Pneumatic Institute to provide such treatments. By the mid-nineteenth century, breathing both oxygen and nitrous oxide had become something akin to a parlor sport. One itinerant organizer of these "laughing gas frolics" along the Eastern seaboard of the United States was Samuel Colt, who controlled his own levity sufficiently to develop the firearm that bears his name.

Ventilatory therapeutics was established on a sound basis near the beginning of the twentieth century. World Wars I and II helped to accelerate interest in developing methods of respiratory augmentation, giving rise to the use of oxygen through a variety of techniques to combat the effects of gas poisoning in World War I and to the development during World War II of high-altitude oxygen masks and demand-breathing valves—the precursors of present clinical ventilators.

PROFESSIONAL HISTORY

At this point the development of respiratory therapy as an allied health profession will be outlined. A regularly scheduled series of lectures that was begun in the Chicago area in the mid-1940s dealt with correct respiratory therapeutic practice, and this series, in cooperation with interested practitioners from New York, culminated in the formation of the Inhalation Therapy Association. In 1950 the Committee on Public Health Relations of the New York Academy of Medicine published standards for inhalation therapy. In 1954 the Inhalation Therapy Association, under the sponsorship of the American College of Chest Physicians (ACCP) and the American Society of Anesthesiologists (ASA), became the American Association of Inhalation Thera-

---

*From Priestley, J.: Experiments and observations on different kinds of air, London, 1775, J. Johnson, vol. 2.

pists. In 1967 this was changed to the American Association for Inhalation Therapy (AAIT), which was modified in 1972 to the American Association for Respiratory Therapy (AART), perhaps from the belated recognition that people exhale as well as inhale!

The profession has continued to develop in cooperation with other closely related professional organizations. The National Board for Respiratory Therapy, founded in 1960 in Illinois as the American Registry of Inhalation Therapists (ARIT) and now known as the American Registry of Respiratory Therapists (ARRT), is an organization committed to achieving the highest standards of technical practice through education and the development of examination procedures for respiratory therapists and respiratory therapy technicians. These two

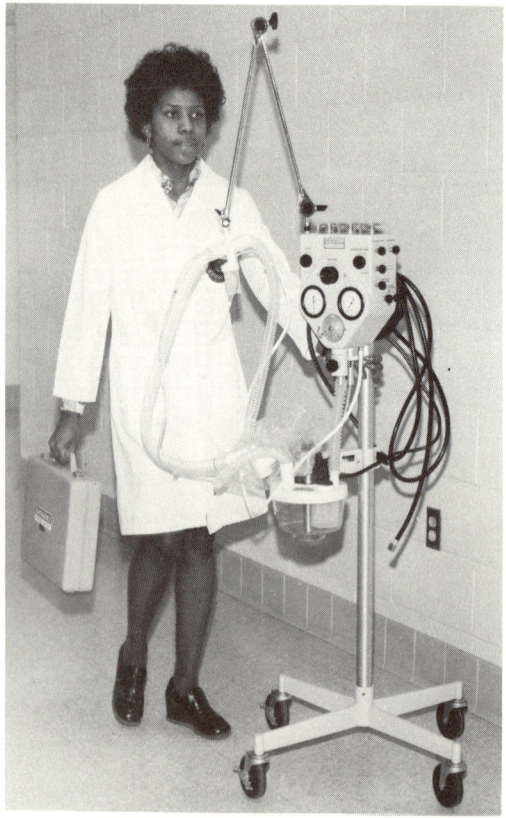

Fig. 32. Prompt provision of a mechanical ventilator in the event of ventilatory failure is one aspect of the respiratory therapist's contribution to coordinated patient care.

principal types of respiratory therapy professionals will be discussed later in this chapter. In 1962 the first edition of what has developed into *Essentials of an Approved Education Program for the Respiratory Therapy Technician and the Respiratory Therapist* was published under the aegis of the Council on Medical Education of the AMA. These criteria have been subsequently revised.

From a struggling organization twenty years ago but with taproots extending back centuries, respiratory therapy has become a vigorous allied health profession of more than 15,000 practitioners, more than 2,500 of whom are registered in their field. Many other practitioners have become certified. The former appellations "tank jockeys" and "oxygen orderlies" are history, and the respiratory therapist—member of a profession that continues to develop—has emerged as a trusted member of the health care team. (See Fig. 32.)

SCOPE OF PROFESSIONAL SERVICES

The functions of the contemporary respiratory therapist may be better understood by considering the services that respiratory therapy is able to offer to the members of one hypothetical family, the Hendersons.

Jimmy Henderson, a premature newborn infant at Children's Hospital, required the prolonged and intensive assistance of the respiratory care service. The drama began in the delivery room where the obstetrician resuscitated Jimmy by using a mask and collapsible oxygen bag; similar in design to those used by respiratory therapists when they regularly participate as members of the hospital's resuscitation team. Jimmy continued to exhibit labored and irregular breathing even after he was placed in an incubator, an apparatus permitting control of the temperature, humidity, and oxygen concentration of an infant's environment.

The respiratory therapist repeatedly obtained and analyzed samples of the infant's blood for oxygen and carbon dioxide partial pressures and noted that the level of carbon dioxide in Jimmy's blood was increasing. The attending physician then ordered that the infant be connected to a ventilator, a mechanical device that provides a variety of breathing patterns to the patient, thereby ensuring more efficient and less tiring ventilation. The respiratory care service worked closely with nursing and medical personnel in observing Jimmy's progress and manipulating the ventilator as required. After six days the ventilator was no longer necessary, and the remainder of Jimmy's hospital stay was uneventful.

Deborah, the Hendersons' younger child, was born three years ago. Delivery was normal, but shortly after birth, she exhibited a slight degree of respiratory distress. At the obstetrician's order she was placed in an incubator. The respiratory therapist, in cooperation with the attending nurses, adjusted the unit to provide the slight increase in oxygen that had been prescribed. By means of an oxygen analyzer, a member of the respiratory care service checked and recorded the oxygen level initially once each half hour and then once every two hours thereafter throughout the several days that Deborah spent in the incubator.

152 Introduction to health professions

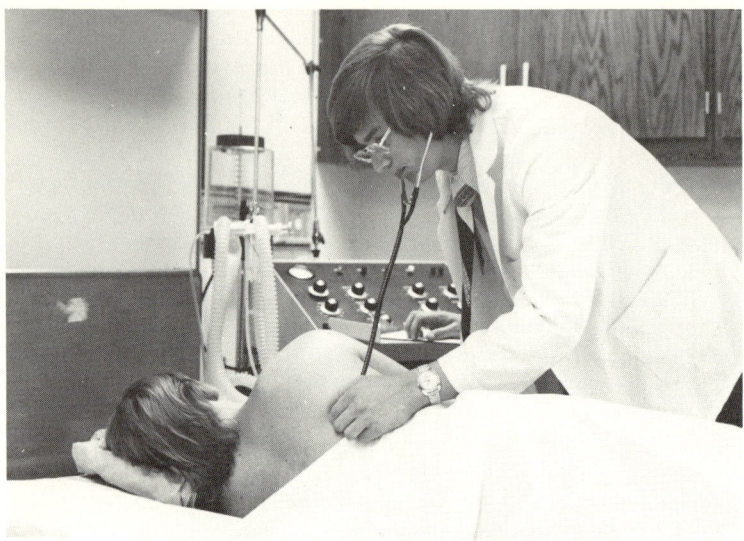

Fig. 33. A respiratory technologist monitors the condition of a drug overdose patient whose respiration is being assisted by a mechanical ventilator.

The use of the manual resuscitation device, the mechanical ventilator, and the blood gas analyzer all have parallels in the techniques that respiratory therapists use to assist adult patients. Doug Henderson, Jimmy and Deborah's father, recently underwent surgery for removal of a lung tumor. His physician, aware that many patients of this type suffer postoperative respiratory complications, contacted the respiratory care service at Community General Hospital. He requested that, in cooperation with the physical therapy department, Mr. Henderson be given preoperative instructions about proper coughing techniques and possible intermittent mechanical ventilation. After his surgery Mr. Henderson developed an elevated temperature, and a chest film taken by the radiologic technologist showed atelectasis, or airlessness, of certain lung areas. Mr. Henderson's physician, judging that an intermittent positive pressure breathing device might cause the affected lung portions to reexpand, ordered it administered in conjunction with mucus-liquefying agents on an hourly basis by the respiratory therapist. Although no dramatic claims were made for the treatment, it is possible that the resources of the respiratory care service and the skill of its staff contributed to the improvement in Mr. Henderson's condition and to decreasing the length of his hospital stay.

The profession's growing involvement in the general community was used to good effect by Frank Henderson, Doug Henderson's father. The area chapter of the American Association for Respiratory Therapy had arranged and staffed a community pulmonary screening program in cooperation with the local lung association and the chest physicians' society. Doug Henderson encouraged his father to go because the senior

Mr. Henderson had complained for some time of being short of breath, and he had a cough that he had come to accept as normal—perhaps as the result of a lifetime of smoking. The respiratory therapist working in the program calculated the readings of Frank Henderson's ability to breath efficiently, as recorded on a device called a spirometer. When the doctor in charge interpreted these records he found indications that Mr. Henderson might be suffering from an obstructive lung disorder. Mr. Henderson was referred to Community General Hospital's outpatient respiratory service. Here the respiratory therapist, working with other health team members, used sophisticated laboratory procedures to carefully assess Mr. Henderson's condition. The respiratory therapist then instructed him in the use of inhaled aerosolized medications, appropriate personal care, and exercises intended to enhance his physical condition. Frank Henderson's lungs will never regain the efficiency they possessed prior to the short-sighted satisfaction of those early cigarettes, but, partly because of the expertise of the respiratory therapist, he now leads a more pleasant life than he had known for many years.

This family vignette illustrates more than a dozen aspects of the routine activities of therapists working in an up-to-the-minute respiratory care service. (See Fig. 33.)

PROFESSIONAL LEVELS AND EDUCATION

Respiratory therapy requires different types of personnel with varying levels of training and preparation, including respiratory therapy assistants, respiratory therapy technicians, and respiratory therapists. Respiratory therapy assistants or aides receive on-the-job training at hospitals that are able to support effective programs of in-service education. Inexperienced personnel are hired as trainees and learn to perform the duties of respiratory therapy assistants. During their training they are also paid employees. Many people presently active in the field began in just this way, although in recent years other avenues have opened for those interested in professional advancement. Respiratory therapy technicians are usually personnel who have completed an AMA-approved educational program designed also to prepare them to apply for certification by the National Board for Respiratory Therapy prior to their employment.

Respiratory therapists must successfully complete a rigorous course of study, also through an AMA-approved program. Such a curriculum is most often based at either a two- or four-year college or university. In addition to the normally required liberal arts studies, the following types of courses are included: basic science, technical theory and its application to various medical specialties, and clinical practice under supervision. For example, a student may study the principles of fluid mechanics in a physics course, examine their application in the interface between a human lung system and a mechanical ventilator, and further observe and practice clinical application in work with pulmonary patients, both medical and surgical.

The prospective student may select one of approximately 120 schools whose programs have received AMA approval. Other schools are presently involved in the approval process. Approximately 5% of the programs offer a B.S. degree. These latter programs not only offer a broad technical and scientific foundation but also prepare interested students for careers in teaching, research, or administration in related fields and provide the groundwork for graduate study in these areas. Requirements for admission vary among schools, but the community college–affiliated programs in particular offer extremely reasonable entrance requirements consistent with their open-door admissions policies. Students are more readily accepted into a program if they have a good science background as well as a high school diploma.

EMPLOYMENT OPPORTUNITIES

At the present time, graduates in respiratory therapy are most likely to locate (after a one-year period of professional employment that separates their actual graduation from the time when they take the national registration or certification examination) in a general or pediatric hospital facility, where they work in either the respiratory therapy department, a pulmonary laboratory setting, or both. Increasingly, however, well-qualified therapists are preparing themselves to enter the ranks of technical educators. The range of vocational opportunities for persons technically competent in matters of respiratory dysfunction is certainly still growing.

Although salaries vary from region to region, the newly graduated respiratory therapist may reasonably expect to begin employment at a salary comparable to or greater than that of a graduate nurse. The registered respiratory therapist may initially receive more than $9,000 annually, and the certified respiratory therapy technician somewhat less.

SUMMARY

This has been a brief look at a young and vigorously growing allied medical profession. As problems of human interaction with the respirable environment continue to mount, this new type of technologist will continue to meet the challenge.

REFERENCE

Priestley, J.: Experiments and observations on different kinds of air, London, 1775, J. Johnson, vol. 2.

SUGGESTED READINGS

Collins, V. J.: Inhalation therapy education and programs, Journal of the American Medical Association **207:** 329, 1969.

Egan, D. F.: Inhalation therapy department: staffing and services, Hospitals **42:**40, 1968.

Egan, D. F.: Fundamentals of respiratory therapy, ed. 2, St. Louis, 1973, The C. V. Mosby Co.

Eisenberg, L.: History of inhalation therapy equipment, International Anesthesiology Clinics **4:**549, 1966.

Gingrich, G. D.: Inhalation therapy service, Hospital Management **107:** 36, 55, 1969.

Miller, W. F.: Respiratory therapy: what does it offer? Anesthesia and Analgesia **47:**599, 1968.

Petty, T. L., and Nett, L. M.: For those who live and breathe, ed. 2, Springfield, Ill., 1972, Charles C Thomas, Publisher.

Respiratory Care, published monthly by the American Association for Respiratory Therapy.

PROFESSIONAL ORGANIZATIONS WHERE FURTHER INFORMATION CAN BE OBTAINED

American Association for Respiratory Therapy
7411 Hines Place
Dallas, Texas 75235

Chapter 22

Social work

Medical social work
Mae M. Davis

Patients who are not overburdened by social, financial, and emotional problems are very often the patients who respond best to medical treatment. A patient who fears the loss of a job requiring maximum physical effort because he has suffered damage to his heart, a mother who frets because she has had to leave her young children while she is confined to a hospital, a diabetic patient who has depended on restaurants for most of his meals and who must now adhere to a restricted diet, a paraplegic whose family must adjust to her doing household tasks from a wheelchair—whatever the nature of the problem, if it is severe enough to retard recovery and lengthen the period of convalescence, the services of the medical social worker are needed. In cases such as these, this highly trained professional becomes an integral part of the patient's total treatment. (See Fig. 34.)

PROFESSIONAL DEVELOPMENT

By the turn of the century, certain physicians had become increasingly aware that social factors play an important role in the cause and treatment of diseases. This awareness led in part to the establishment of medical social work as a specialty in the field of social work at Massachusetts General Hospital in Boston in 1905. By 1910 the New York School of Social Work, in cooperation with Bellevue Hospital in New York City, developed a major course of study for hospital social service workers. The role of the medical social worker has evolved from these pioneering efforts in Boston and New York.

In the course of its development the social work profession has used many different approaches in working with the various elements of human society—family, community, and ethnic or racial groups—and with the relationships and institutions involved in daily life and well-being. Medical social work has traditionally been concerned with the individual who has been moved from his family setting to the confines of a hospital or institution because of an illness. Through various changes in role, the medical social worker has become actively engaged in helping to extend the concept of medical care beyond the walls of the hospital. Medical social work traditionally dealt only with stresses in the crisis situation of hospitalization. Today it is involved with pro-

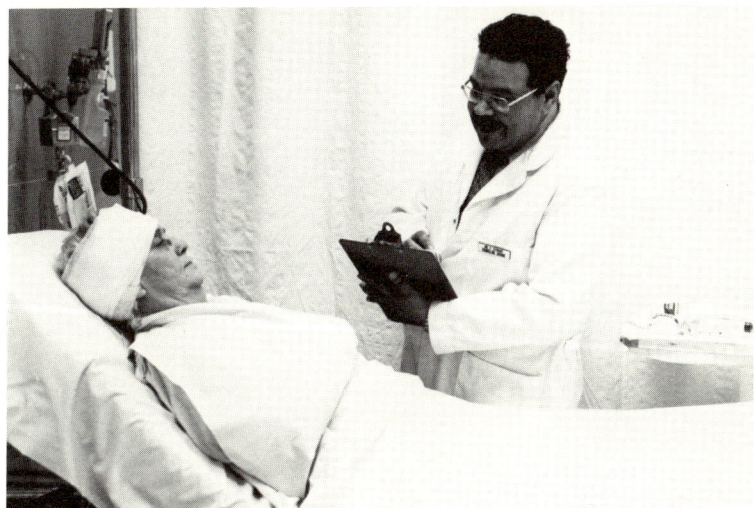

Fig. 34. A woman treated in the emergency room for multiple injuries resulting from a car accident discusses with a medical social worker the need for planning care for her aged mother who will be alone at home.

gramming health care to help prevent breakdowns in social function and promote rehabilitation.

EDUCATIONAL REQUIREMENTS

Medical social service departments within hospitals carry out their programs of helping patients through professional standards of practice. In order to maintain these standards, directors of medical social service departments must hold master's degrees in social work. Such departments usually hire staff social workers with master's degrees and assistant social workers with bachelor's degrees in social welfare from colleges and universities accredited by the Council on Social Work Education.

Master's and doctor's degrees are awarded for advanced study to students who have demonstrated their abilities in supervisory and leadership roles in a number of practice areas in the field of social work. Undergraduate programs in social work or social welfare are now offered by more than 200 colleges. The number of schools whose curriculums are accredited by the Council on Social Work Education is steadily increasing. The bachelor's degree is accepted as the initial certificate for professional practice in social work. In 1970, graduates of baccalaureate programs in social work became eligible to apply for regular membership in the National Association of Social Workers. Those with a bachelor's degree in such related fields as sociology, psychology, or education who are currently employed in social work agencies may apply for an associate membership.

Candidates for the baccalaureate degree must meet the college or university's basic requirements for course work in the arts and sciences. Usually students must complete courses in the social sciences, the natural sciences, and the humanities and take courses concerned with the development of basic reading, writing, and verbal communication skills. Typical requirements include a selection of courses in such areas as anthropology, biology, geology, zoology, philosophy, sociology, psychology, history, certain foreign languages, and English. The student majoring in social work follows a course sequence for the first two years that is approved by the department or school of social work.

Curriculum requirements for the junior and senior years consist essentially of courses in social work, sociology, and choices from a specified group of electives. These are typically concentrated in such areas as social systems, social policy, criminology, social factors in personality, race relations, juvenile delinquency, behavior and social movements, sociology of urban life, social welfare and human needs, and government social welfare programs and policies. In their senior year, students are assigned to social agencies, health agencies, hospitals, schools, and other institutions so that they can observe professionals at work and acquire supervised experience. Students who want to specialize in medical social work must earn their bachelor's and master's degrees and complete a period of professionally supervised experience in a hospital or health care facility. In other words, the medical specialization is not offered in either graduate or undergraduate social work programs.

PROFESSIONAL FUNCTIONS

Professional social work is the art and science concerned with meeting and satisfying human and social needs. It is directed toward serving both individuals and the society in which they live. Social workers achieve their objectives by working with individuals, families, and the community. Medical social workers usually work in situations where individuals are confined to hospitals or are being treated in clinics for illness or injury. The medical social worker employs two primary skills in working with patients: the art of listening and the art of establishing a carefully and consciously developed relationship. Data are gathered for every patient and developed into a medical-social history for the use of physicians and other members of the patient care team who participate in treatment and planning. Medical social work may involve not only interviews with the patient but also consultation with family members, friends, employers, teachers, and ministers as well as with personnel from other hospitals and health care and social service agencies. It involves referrals to service agencies in the community where various kinds of follow-up help are available to the patient after his discharge from the hospital. Hospital medical social workers may continue to serve a former patient in outpatient clinics and through home visits. Medical social work requires contact with the patient's physician, skill in reading medical chart progress records, and an understanding of medical terminology relating to treatment procedures and medical-surgical diagnoses. At times the medical social worker must interpret a diagnosis and its significance to the patient, his family, and other social workers in the community who may also become involved.

The following account illustrates the activities of a medical social worker.*

> Mrs. S., 30 years of age, a registered nurse and mother of four children, was referred to the caseworker at the time her 3-year-old daughter Cheryl had an eye removed because of a tumor behind the eyeball. The prognosis for Cheryl was poor.
>
> The reason for the referral was that Mrs. S., experiencing conflict about her roles as nurse and mother, had exhibited explosive behavior on the ward. As a nurse she was able to understand the seriousness of her daughter's illness but found it hard to accept because the onset had been so sudden, and because she had considered Cheryl to be the healthiest, brightest, and most outgoing of her four children.
>
> At the outset she resented the referral but the caseworker was able to convince her that the staff was genuinely interested in helping her and recognized that she was upset with good reason. The worker also pointed out that frequently professional people find it difficult to maintain an objective attitude when they attempt to assist family members with whom they are emotionally involved. She was then able to appraise her actions, to be less critical of the nursing staff, and to turn over the responsibilities for the child's care to them. Her relationship with members of the medical staff also improved.
>
> In the meantime, neighbors in the close-knit community in which the family resided had rallied behind the family and were helping to care for the children at home, thus enabling their father to resume working as an engineer with an aircraft firm. Mrs. S. was grateful for the assistance but distressed that it was necessary. The worker helped her to see that the neighbors were glad to be helpful and that she should accept the help in the spirit in which it was given.
>
> Mrs. S. became increasingly able to handle her anxieties but was concerned about her husband who, she felt, was having trouble in facing the seriousness of Cheryl's illness. In a lengthy discussion with the caseworker, Mr. S. expressed anger toward the doctors because he felt there had been too long a delay before the surgery was performed. The worker was able to show him that his anger toward the medical staff was related to his own frustration and helplessness in the situation. She suggested that he express his feelings to the chief resident as he was the one who had followed Cheryl through all her hospitalizations, and she

---

*Adapted from Kennedy, N.: Helping the dying patient and his family, New York, 1960, Family Service Association of America.

arranged such a meeting. She also told him about his wife's concern for him. Mrs. S. later reported that the interview had helped them both and that they were reaching toward each other for needed support and comfort.

Cheryl's condition continued to decline and during the last few days preceding her death, the caseworker talked frequently with the parents, encouraging them to express their feelings and discussing with them how they might best prepare the other children. Both parents took their daughter's death quite well. The caseworker continued counseling Mrs. S. who with her children remained under Medical Center care for several months.

In summary, the worker felt that although Mrs. S. had been initially resistive to the referral, she was able to use the help given, not only in relation to facing Cheryl's illness and death but in relation to other problem areas. She evidenced good ego strength and became able to handle subsequent crisis situations such as a possible neurological disorder in the oldest child which was later ruled out. After eight months, when no further problems had arisen, the case was closed.

FURTHER SCOPE OF RESPONSIBILITY

Medical social workers are responsible for keeping adequate records of the services rendered to every patient. They are required to attend various medical and surgical conferences with groups of physicians, nurses, and other health professionals to discuss patient situations and to plan for the best follow-up patient care. Their responsibilities may also involve budget and financial assistance planning with patients and their families to ensure their having adequate housing, medicines, equipment such as a wheelchair and hospital bed, transportation to and from the clinic or doctor's office, and adequate food and clothing.

CAREER OPPORTUNITIES

This has been only a brief overview of the many services rendered by the medical social worker in a hospital. It should be remembered that these professionals also perform their services in various health agencies, welfare departments, extended care facilities, nursing homes, and other patient care institutions.

There are numerous professional opportunities in medical social work, and indeed in all fields of social work, both in government and in private settings. Approximately 175,000 job openings in the 1970s were predicted from 1965 studies made by the United States Department of Labor. There are many opportunities available in specialized areas such as psychiatric programs for the mentally ill or mentally retarded, children's and family services, adoption services, mental health programs, rehabilitation, government welfare programs, and services to the aged, blind, crippled, and disabled. Many volunteer organizations such as the Epilepsy Association, American Cancer

Society, American Heart Association, the Kidney Foundation, the Arthritis Foundation, and their state and local auxiliary organizations also employ medical social workers.

The National Association of Social Workers, Inc., through its Committee on Professional Standards and Practice, has established salary standards that are based on the social worker's academic training and experience. Geographic area, economic stresses, and the sources of revenue for agencies' support influence the amounts expended for social workers' salaries. During 1975, professionally qualified social workers with the bachelor's degree should find that salaries range from $8,000 to $10,000 annually; with the master's degree, annual salaries range from $10,500 to $13,500.

SUMMARY

Medical social workers are experts in the field of human relations, trained to understand people and their needs. They use their knowledge, skills, and judgment to help the patient and his family handle their social, emotional, and financial problems. In addition, they must have a thorough knowledge of the community resources that are available to aid the troubled patient and his family. The medical social worker needs objectivity and good judgment in order to view all facets of human problems with warm and compassionate understanding from a practical and realistic perspective.

Social work in mental health settings
Elizabeth J. Laschinger

The purpose of professional social workers is the improvement of their clients' abilities to (1) meet the challenges of their lives, (2) solve the problems of living with themselves and other people, and (3) prevent the occurrence of problems in the future. Professional social workers help people to understand themselves, their feelings, their relationships with other people, and to use themselves and the people around them so that living is more understandable, more fulfilling, and more satisfying.

Mental health settings are places in which care and treatment are provided to people of all ages who are troubled or disturbed. These settings include public and private psychiatric hospitals, psychiatric units of general hospitals, day treatment centers, and public and private clinics.

Because there is much to be learned about how the mind and emotions affect behavior, mental health settings usually employ people with knowledge and skills from many disciplines. There may be psychiatrists, educators, clinical psychologists, social workers, vocational counselors, nurses, occupational therapists, and others—all of whom have specialized in understanding the mentally and emotionally ill.

PROFESSIONAL FUNCTIONS

Professional social workers in these settings are frequently asked to help the "therapeutic team" understand those aspects of the patient's world around him (environment) that are of help to him, those that are damaging to him, and those that are of no use. Other team members may be working to answer such questions as: "What sort of a person is this individual? Are there physical reasons for his behavior? How does he cope with life? What are his strengths? His weaknesses?" Together the team tries to understand why an individual feels and functions as he does and what can be done to help him. The helping process may include individual or group psychotherapy, the use of psychotherapeutic drugs, effecting a change in the way family members feel and act toward each other, education and job planning with the patient and community, his removal from an environment in which he cannot cope, and many other possible alternatives. Social work involves most of these treatment aspects.

In the past, "treatment" of the seriously disturbed adult offered few alternatives to months or years of custodial care in a mental hospital. The professional social worker's responsibilities were limited frequently to making arrangements for food, clothing, and shelter for those comparatively few patients who could leave the hospital. Little by little, new knowledge about mental illness and how to treat it emerged, and by the 1940s professional social workers were being asked to engage in intensive counseling. This required that social workers gain greater knowledge and deeper understanding of the reasons for and causes of mental illness and emotional pain. Because professional social workers use themselves as instruments of helping, it was necessary that they gain a greater understanding of their "use of self"—how their beliefs and biases, values, and attitudes about people helped or hindered them in their work of helping people effect change in themselves.

By the 1960s a number of psychotherapeutic medicines were available and aided many of the mentally ill and emotionally disturbed to feel better about themselves, and enabled them to act responsibly and more effectively in the complex world outside the hospital. At the same time, community mental health centers were being established not only to keep people from getting so sick that hospitalization would be required but also to help others who were feeling overwhelmed by the pain that feelings can cause.

For years, professional social workers had been serving families in other social work settings such as public and private family and children's agencies. Their acquired knowledge and experience had developed ways of helping whole families, rather than just one member, when the family was "falling apart." As social workers moved to the community mental health centers, their knowledge and skills in family therapy were employed in these new settings.

SOCIAL WORK CLASSIFICATION

In 1973 the National Association of Social Workers published *Standards for Social Service Manpower*, which sets forth the following six-level classification.

Preprofessional

Social service aide   no educational requirements, entry based on individual's personal qualifications and employment in a social agency

Social service technician   completion of a two-year junior or community college education in one of the social services, with an associate arts or baccalaureate degree in another field

Professional

Social worker   a baccalaureate degree from an accredited program

Graduate social worker   a master's degree from an accredited graduate school of social work

Certified social worker   certification by the Academy of Certified Social Workers (ACSW) as being capable of the autonomous, self-directed practice of social work

Social work fellow   completion of a doctoral program or substantial practice in the field of specialization following certification by ACSW

EDUCATIONAL REQUIREMENTS AND CAREER OPPORTUNITIES

Social workers at all professional levels are employed in community mental health centers. Mental health aides and technicians perform helping tasks. Professional social workers with a bachelor's degree may counsel individuals, families, and small groups of distressed people, often with another professional person as "co-therapist." Social workers with more education and skill may work as more skilled counselors; as educators and supervisors to less experienced staff members; as consultants in mental health to schools, businesses, and other health and social agencies; as researchers in mental health and community problems; and as administrators of the center's services.

Mental hospitals also employ social workers at all professional levels. Those holding a bachelor's degree assist patients in making living arrangements after they leave the hospital (housing, income, and activities) and in planning for the other help they may need in terms of outpatient or community mental health services.

Mental health services for children through the years have made extensive use of professional social workers in hospitals and institutions for distrubed children and in child guidance clinics. Mental health services to children are not presently as widely available as those for adults, but such programs as Headstart (educational opportunities for the underprivileged preschool child), private family agencies, and federal, state, and county programs in child welfare do provide the knowledgeable help of social workers to many distressed children and their families.

SUMMARY

A career in professional social work begins with the acquisition of a bachelor's degree from a college or university whose social work program is accredited by the Council of Social Work Education. This education provides the basic core of knowledge, the techniques of helping people with social problems, and an understanding of how to use oneself to help people change. Graduate education provides increased knowledge and skills as a clinician, supervisor, administrator, community researcher, or planner. Professional social workers direct their altruistic concern, compassionate commitment, and open desire for further knowledge toward helping people to live with themselves and others in more fulfilling relationships.

REFERENCES

Bartlett, H.: The common base of social work practice, Washington, D.C., 1970, National Association of Social Workers, Inc.

Encyclopedia of Social Work, Washington, D.C., 1971, National Association of Social Workers, Inc.

Ferguson, E. A.: Social work, an introduction, ed. 3, Philadelphia, 1975, J. B. Lippincott Co.

Kennedy, N.: Helping the dying patient and his family, New York, 1960, Family Service Association of America.

Perlman, H. H.: Persona–social role and personality, Chicago, 1968, The University of Chicago Press.

Standards for social service manpower, Washington, D.C., 1973, National Association of Social Workers, Inc.

SUGGESTED READINGS

Baker, R. L., and Briggs, T. L.: Differential use of social work manpower, New York, 1968, National Association of Social Workers, Inc.

Perlman, H. H., editor: Helping—Charlotte Towle on social work and social casework, Chicago, 1969, The University of Chicago Press.

PROFESSIONAL ORGANIZATIONS WHERE FURTHER INFORMATION CAN BE OBTAINED

National Association of Social Workers, Inc.
600 Southern Building
15th and H Streets
Washington, D.C. 20005

Council on Social Work Education
345 East 46th Street
New York, New York 10017

Chapter 23

Speech and hearing science

John W. Black

WHAT IS SPEECH AND HEARING SCIENCE?

Speech and hearing science is neither new nor narrow in scope. It deals with the system people use for verbal communication. Conversation, public speeches, acting, or reading aloud are all means of communicating, whether the parties are face to face or use electronic equipment. It is acoustic, involving talking and listening. These systems are so important that persons with defective speech or hearing are often treated at public expense. Moses lamented, "I am slow of speech," and commonly special reference is made to a person's speech skills. For example, letters of recommendation often include comments on the manner in which a person communicates and refer to the quality of voice, articulation, pronunciation, and vocabulary. (See Fig. 35.)

Specialists in speech and hearing science may be referred to as speech and hearing therapists, speech pathologists and audiologists, logopedists, or phoniatrists. They have studied such topics as (1) speech and hearing disorders; (2) the development of language; (3) the development of language processes in children; (4) language and speech for the deaf; (5) vocal pitch, loudness, and quality; (6) the physics (acoustics) of speech; (7) the anatomy and physiology of the head and neck and the process of respiration; (8) the theories and measurement of hearing; (9) semantics; and (10) phonetics.

Speech and hearing scientists do not work alone. They are part of a team whose members vary according to the special needs of each patient or client. Team members may be teachers, medical specialists (pediatricians, surgeons, otologists, neurologists, physiatrists, and psychiatrists), dental specialists, psychologists, nurses, and social workers. The typical specialist in speech and hearing works with other professional people and serves individuals of all ages.

In hospital settings, speech and hearing specialists see patients recovering from laryngectomies or surgical repair of cleft palates. They may also work with those who are considering an operation on the middle ear as well as those who have Parkinson's disease or who have suffered a stroke. In schools they often work with children who talk with obvious misarticulations, stutter, have voice disorders or a loss of hearing, or are slow in developing language skills. In clinics, speech and hearing specialists deal with all of these types of disorders in ad-

166 Introduction to health professions

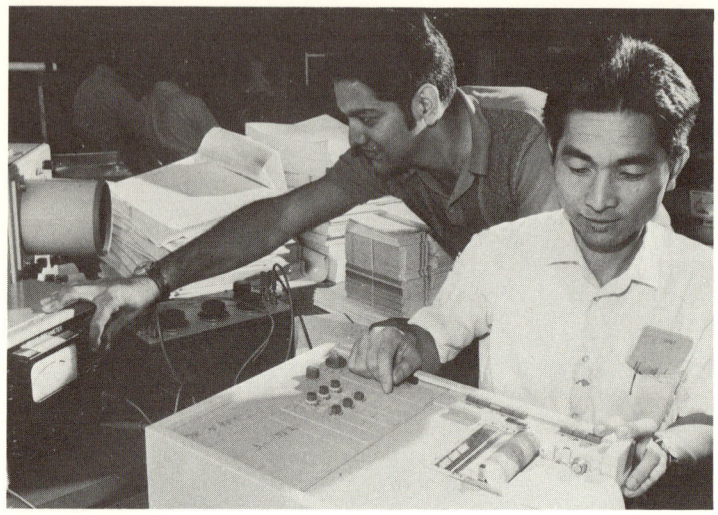

Fig. 35. Speech and hearing scientists are studying the intonation patterns of some well-known speakers for research purposes.

dition to working with persons who seek assistance in learning to communicate more effectively. In industry they may assess the hearing of employees who work in an environment where there are high noise levels. They may work in laboratories to improve hearing aids and telephones or design electronic devices that people can use for self-instruction.

WHAT IS THE HISTORY OF SPEECH AND HEARING SCIENCE?

Speech and hearing science has been the subject of much study. In 1779 the annual prize of the Russian Academy of Science was awarded for an explanation and successful simulation of vowel sounds. Although Alexander Graham Bell is best known for his work on the telephone, this invention evolved from his achievements as a phonetician (a student of speech sounds) and his work in teaching deaf persons to communicate. His interest in the field had been spurred by his wife's acute hearing loss. Sir Richard Paget, an Englishman with interests similar to Bell's, served as President of the British Deaf and Dumb Association and wrote an especially scholarly account of a theory of the origin of language, a work that contrasts sharply with Bell's phonetics books and inventions with their practical applications. Professor Edward Scripture was absorbed with the same core of facts that intrigued Bell and Paget. He worked first as an experimental psychologist and subsequently as a theoretical and practical speech pathologist. Scripture's works related primarily to talking rather than hearing and illustrate the diversity among speech and language pathologists and audiologists, or speech and hearing scientists. Harvey Fletcher began his career in speech and hearing science as a physicist in a university. His interests expanded in many directions as he coped with the topics of telephony in the Bell Telephone Laboratories. The insights of this distinguished researcher extended the horizons of speech and hearing science. Herman Helmholtz, an eminent German psychologist and physicist, maintained an active interest in hearing. His monumental volume, *The Sensation of Tone*, is available to students of speech and hearing science in a highly readable English translation by the dedicated phonetician Alexander J. Ellis, who studied and translated the epoch-making work of Helmholtz in his own search for a rationale for the perception of speech.

These examples illustrate the many phases of speech and hearing science, or speech and language pathology and audiology. They may clarify why the term "speech and hearing scientist" is used in this chapter to represent the fully trained practitioner-teacher-researcher, the product of sustained undergraduate, graduate, and professional specialization.

WHAT ARE THE CRITERIA OF ADEQUATE VOICE COMMUNICATION?

From the point of view of speech and hearing science, the following principal criteria are used to evaluate the communication system: (1) intelligibility both in talking and in hearing, (2) pleasantness of voice and minimal distraction in the production of speech, and (3) an adequate vocabulary and use of correct syntax.

Intelligibility can be graded, that is, given a numerical score. Intelligibility depends on the speaker, the listener, the acoustics of the room in which the speaking takes place, and the unit at a person's ear; for example, a telephone receiver or a hearing aid.

Pleasantness in speech is first an absence of certain readily identifiable vocal qualities, rhythms, and patterns of pitch that are identified with speech disorders. Reducing the distracting movements and mannerisms that may accompany abnormal talking has more than just cosmetic value.

The language that is used in talking is evaluated at all ages. Is this child developing normally? Can this patient make sense? Can either one of them understand me? Here the topic is normal versus abnormal speech and language. The professional worker must also be interested in the adequacy of speech skills for special uses. For example, a person who is employing a sales clerk, receptionist, or telephone operator needs people whose speech will be effective in those situations.

WHAT ARE THE NEEDS FOR PROFESSIONAL SPEECH AND HEARING SCIENTISTS?

Because speech and hearing skills affect our public as well as our private lives, the shortage of people who are trained to work with speech and hearing is especially critical. This shortage affects universities, state and local health agencies, and schools, and accordingly there is an increasing use of supportive personnel such as hospital corpsmen trained in audiology who work with speech pathologists and audiologists.

Training programs for supportive personnel are only now being developed. The laws in some states permit agencies to sponsor in-service programs to train high school graduates as audiometrists. Some universities are also experimenting with brief courses of study to train aides who will work routinely with isolated segments of speech therapy.

HOW DOES ONE STUDY SPEECH AND HEARING SCIENCE?

Speech and hearing science may be taught in university or college departments established to deal with these areas, or relevant courses may be offered in a number of departments involved with different subjects related to speech and hearing.

Undergraduate students majoring in speech and hearing science study voice and diction, acoustics, phonetics, speech development in children, anatomy and physiology of the ear and vocal mechanisms, and introductory speech pathology and audiology. They study psychology and should include courses in languages, linguistics, anthropology, mathematics, and biology in their undergraduate programs. This course work constitutes preprofessional study.

It is important that graduate students clearly keep in mind the professional requirements of the American Speech and Hearing Association. To qualify for a certificate of clinical competence, candidates must meet the following requirements.

1. They must be members of the American Speech and Hearing Association.
2. They must submit transcripts from one or more accredited colleges or universities presenting evidence of the completion of a well-integrated program of sixty semester hours that includes eighteen semester hours in the normal development and use of speech, hearing, and language and forty-two semester hours in the management of speech, hearing, and language disorders and in supplementary or related fields. Of these forty-two semester hours, at least six must be in audiology (for the speech pathologist) or in speech pathology (for the audiologist). No more than six may be in courses that provide academic credit for clinical practice. At least twenty-four semester hours, not including credit for a thesis or dissertation, must be in courses in the field in which certification is being sought. Furthermore, thirty semester hours must be in courses that may be applied

toward a graduate degree by the college or university at which these courses are taken.
3. They must submit evidence of the completion of 300 clock hours of supervised, direct clinical experience in working with individuals who have a variety of communication disorders. This experience must be obtained within the training institution or in one of its cooperating programs, and more than half of this experience must be obtained during graduate study.
4. They must also present written references from employers and supervisors of nine months of full-time professional employment in the area in which certification is being sought.
5. Finally, candidates must pass a nationally administered written examination.

Simultaneously with their professional study, prospective specialists master the tools of research and independent study to enable them to approach a client in the spirit of inquiry rather than prescription. They read the professional literature with understanding and seek to make their own contributions to it.

Much of the student's practical experience is gained through work in a speech and hearing clinic. Typical university clinics offer four types of interrelated services.
1. They provide opportunities for prospective professionals in public schools, colleges, hospitals, community agencies, private clinics, or private practice to work with and observe clinical cases.
2. They provide clinical cases for original study and research in speech and hearing disorders.
3. They extend free services to university students who have impaired hearing or speech deviations.
4. They render services in speech correction and hearing disorders to members of the general community. (See Fig. 36.)

The typical university clinic is coordinated by a director or supervisor, who accepts cases for examination and therapy in keeping with the four purposes of the clinic and according to its best interest. The director maintains and preserves a record on each person who is accepted for examination or therapy. Such clinics handle a variety of cases such as the following.
1. *Speech:* Each client is given a speech evaluation, and recommendations are made. Most therapy is individual. When there are a sufficient number of persons with a similar defect, supplemental clinics are organized for corrective group instruction. The following types of groups may be formed:
   a. Children 3 to 4 years of age (preschoolers) with delayed language development
   b. Children 5 to 8 years of age with delayed speech or language problems
   c. Children 5 to 8 years of age with articulation difficulties

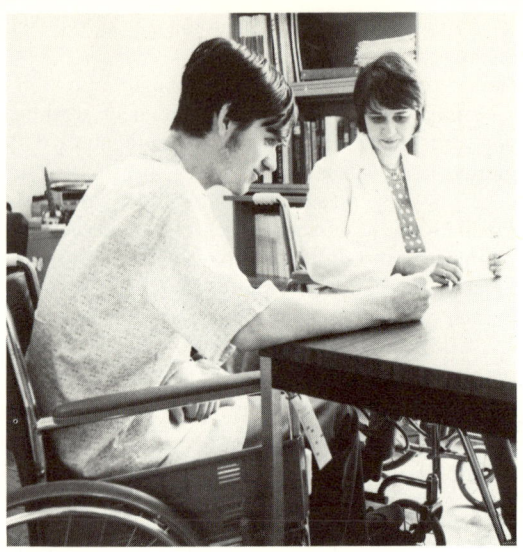

Fig. 36. A speech pathologist in a rehabilitation center helps a client to relearn language skills.

    d. Children who stutter
    e. Children with repaired palates
    f. Stutterers 10 to 16 years of age
    g. Adult stutterers
    h. Patients with brain injuries, for example, aphasics
    i. Individuals who have undergone laryngectomies
    j. Persons who speak with foreign dialects
    k. Adults with voice problems
2. *Hearing:* The services include audiometric testing, lipreading (speech reading) instruction, auditory training, speech correction for the articulatory and voice disorders that occur in many instances with a loss of hearing, and hearing aid evaluations.

All services are coordinated with those offered by other members of the allied health professions.

Current salary scales for speech pathologists and audiologists relate closely to the different levels of training and are further contingent on regional cost-of-living indices.

Level of training	Median (beginning) salary (first 9 to 10 months)
Doctoral degree	$12,800
Master's degree	$ 9,500
Bachelor's degree	$ 8,000
Other supportive personnel	$4/5$ of next higher level

• • •

The following case study illustrates the various contributions that speech and hearing scientists can make in evaluating client problems and helping clients to achieve improvements.

Mrs. Burns brought her 7-year-old son Tommy to the University Speech and Hearing Clinic. She explained that Tommy had difficulty in forming "s" sounds, that he was unable to make himself understood, and that he stuttered at times. According to his mother, Tommy's early motor and speech development had been normal. He had just completed the first grade, and he reportedly enjoyed it very much. However, his teacher reported that he confused many words due to his inability to differentiate between many of the sounds in the English language. Because of this difficulty, he was to attend summer school five mornings a week, as his teacher felt this additional stimulation and training period would give him better preparation for the second grade. Tommy has a brother Steven who is 5 years of age. The brothers are quite close and usually play harmoniously together, according to their mother.

Mrs. Burns is divorced and works as a clerk in a department store. While she is at work, her mother babysits with the children. When he stays with his grandmother, Tommy does not receive much stimulation even from children's television programs, since he is permitted to watch only his grandmother's favorite programs. For example, he has never seen "Sesame Street" or any of the shows designed especially to interest youngsters.

Mrs. Burns was 30 years of age when Tommy was born. She reported that hemorrhaging had occurred approximately twenty-four hours before his birth, which was two weeks premature. Although Tommy weighed 8 pounds when he was born, he was placed in an incubator for two weeks.

Mrs. Burns appeared to be an interested, intelligent parent. She realized that Tommy could benefit from greater environmental stimulation and was receptive to the examiner's recommendations for improvement in this area.

A specialized articulation test was administered and Tommy was found to make the following errors:
1. At the beginning of words he would substitute *s* for "ch" and say *soo* for "chew"; substitute *w* for "r" and say *wed* for "red"; substitute *g* for "j," saying *gill* for "jill"; substitute *d* for "th," saying *dough* for "though"; and substitute *d* for "z," saying *dip* for "zip."
2. In the middle of words, Tommy would substitute *k* for "t," saying *kiken* for "kitten"; substitute *s* for "sh," saying *fasin* for "fashion"; substitute *d* for "r," saying *tidesome* for "tiresome"; substitute *h* for "th," say *gaher* for "gather"; and substitute *g* for "z" saying *regen* for "reason."
3. At the end of some words, Tommy would substitute *d* for "r," saying *load* for "lower."

When asked to do so, Tommy was successful in pronouncing *sh, t, ch, z,* and *th* in nonsense syllables such as "sha," "ta," "cha," "za," and "tha"; and there did not seem to be anything wrong with his articulatory mechanism. He could move his tongue at will and had intact teeth, palate, and lips. Pure-tone audiometry tests indicated that his hearing was within normal limits. However, when he was asked to repeat words as he heard them, he made more mistakes than would be expected, missing five of the thirteen items on the Boston University Short Discrimination Test. On a standard test of intelligence, Tommy attained the raw score of 60, a mental age of 6 years and 10 months, and an I.Q. of 89. On the geometric form copying task of this test, Tommy successfully copied the circle, cross, square, and triangle—a performance level appropriate for a child 6 years of age. On the Goodenough Draw-A-Man Test, Tommy's drawing was characteristic of a child 5 years and 9 months of age.

Tommy is right-handed. His performance in hopping on one foot, throwing a ball, running, and rail walking indicated normal gross motor coordination. His manipulation of the pencil for drawing demonstrated normal fine motor coordination. No dysfluencies were noted during the diagnostic evaluation, nor could they be precipitated by increasing communicative stress.

On the basis of these tests and observations, it was concluded that Tommy had a moderate functional articulation problem and poor auditory discrimination skills. It was therefore recommended that he be enrolled for speech therapy, with special emphasis to be placed on building his auditory awareness in general and his auditory discrimination skill in particular. His progress or improvement was to be measured after three months of therapy through administration of the Peabody Picture Vocabulary Test, Form A. Mrs. Burns was advised to check the public library for reading material on speech and language acquisition. Her permission was requested to send the results to Tommy's teacher together with recommendations.

The low level of Tommy's environmental stimulation appears to be a strong etiological factor in his general lack of awareness of sounds and existing differences between sounds. Although he is stimulable for may of his error phonemes, prognosis is only fair due to his distinct deficiency in auditory discrimination.

SUGGESTED READINGS

Davis, H., and Silverman, S. R.: Hearing and deafness, ed. 3, New York, 1970, Holt, Rinehart & Winston, Inc.

Denes, P. B., and Pinson, E. N.: The speech chain, Baltimore, 1963, The Williams & Wilkins Co.

Van Riper, C.: Speech correction: principles and methods, ed. 5, Englewood Cliffs, N.J., 1972, Prentice-Hall, Inc.

Wise, C. M.: Introduction to phonetics, Englewood Cliffs, N.J., 1957, Prentice-Hall, Inc.

PROFESSIONAL ORGANIZATION WHERE FURTHER INFORMATION CAN BE OBTAINED

American Speech and Hearing Association
9030 Old Georgetown Road
Washington, D.C. 20014

Chapter 24
Veterinary medicine
Clarence R. Cole

Veterinary medicine is concerned with the health and well-being of animals and human beings, the control of diseases transmissible from animals to human beings, and the discovery of new knowledge in comparative medicine. It has existed as one of the healing arts since prehistoric people perceived that the health of their animals was nearly as important as their own health. Records of ancient civilizations show some attempt to describe and treat illnesses of animals. Four thousand years ago an Egyptian papyrus recorded prescriptions for diseases of dogs and cows.

HISTORY OF THE PROFESSION

Nearly 200 years ago Benjamin Rush, physician and veterinarian, signer of the Declaration of Independence, and member of the Continental Congress and the medical faculty of the University of Pennsylvania, spoke of there being only one medicine. He was pleading for one of the many causes he championed—the establishment of veterinary medical colleges in the United States. His plea went unanswered for nearly half a century, until the truth of his arguments became all too evident. Disease acquired from animals caused widespread human illness and death, and food shortages resulted from epidemics among food-producing animals. It was a truth that has been demonstrated throughout history. Tuberculosis, rabies, typhus, and many other diseases, some of the most dreaded health threats, are passed from animals to people.

VETERINARY MEDICINE TODAY

Historically, veterinary medicine has come to the rescue of a disappearing food supply. Doctors of veterinary medicine, from those who guard the health of protein-producing farm animals to those who set and enforce standards for pure food from animal sources, monitor the food-processing industry. Safeguarding our food supply by ensuring livestock health and the wholesomeness of foods of animal origin is one of the veterinarian's important functions. Through this work the whole population is served directly.

Modern veterinarians, however, are responsible for a host of other safeguards—both to human and animal health—that are often simply taken for granted as part of the blessings of modern life. The control of rabies is a classical case in point. Anyone who has undergone the painful series of antirabies inoculations and knows that because of them he has been spared far greater suffering and certain death is not likely to dismiss lightly the veterinarian's contribution in this field. Fortunately, few of us fall into this category, thanks to the work of veterinarians. In 1945 over 10,000 cases of rabies in animals were reported, and thousands of people were treated with antirabies serum. There have been only nine reported human deaths from rabies in the United States between 1951 and 1974. Its incidence has been decreased by 76% in the last fifteen years. Yet because rabies still persists in wild animals, veterinarians have the responsibility for vaccinating pets so that they cannot become a link in transmitting the disease from wild animals to human beings.

Because of their special knowledge of diseases that affect both animals and people, the work of veterinarians is essential to the control of zoonoses, one of the greatest concerns in the field of public health. Zoonoses are diseases transmissible from animals to human beings. Rabies is one of the zoonoses that no longer threatens human health because veterinarians have brought it under control in domesticated animals.

In 1893 Dr. Theobald Smith, who was chief pathologist of the United States Bureau of Animal Industry in Washington, D.C., and Dr. F. L. Kilbourne, a veterinarian and director of the Veterinary Experimental Station of the Bureau from 1885 to 1894, published a paper, *Investigations into the Nature, Cause, and Prevention of Texas or Southern Cattle Fever*. In the paper the two doctors furnished the first proof that diseases can be transmitted by insects, something that had not been suspected until shortly before the turn of the century. Their discovery not only led to the eradication of Texas fever but provided the basis for Walter Reed's breakthrough regarding yellow fever in 1900. Other researchers went on to discover the insect links, or "vectors," responsible for transmitting malaria, typhus, African sleeping sickness, and Rocky Mountain spotted fever from their wild animal reservoirs to man.

The list of diseases controlled through the work of veterinarians is impressive and may lull us into thinking that zoonotic study is a closed chapter in medical history. The facts are less reassuring. According to the World Health Organization, 30 of the more than 175 known zoonoses occur with some frequency in the United States. And these may shift insidiously because mutations in microorganisms can cause them to adapt to new hosts, possibly creating new zoonoses. Continual vigilance and alertness are needed to prevent them from becoming threats to human health.

In addition to old enemies in new disguises, diseases that were formerly found only in remote regions are being spread by the increasing convenience, speed, and volume of trade and travel and now are a worldwide threat to animal and human health.

Far from being exclusively concerned with animals, the veterinary medical profession today is oriented toward comparative medicine and the biomedical sciences. The veterinarian is in the forefront of space medicine and marine research, comparative pathology, and efforts to discover new and safe treatments for human and animal diseases.

Nearly all members of the veterinary profession, regardless of the branch of medicine in which they work, encounter disease conditions in animals that can contribute to an understanding of human medical problems. Since veterinary medical training involves many animal species, it provides a particularly good background for studies in comparative medicine.

There are many ways in which veterinarians combat both human and animal illnesses. Animal models of human diseases can be used for experimentation by veterinarians, who are familiar with both the animal and human forms of the disease. For example, swine, pigeons, and monkeys spontaneously develop arteriosclerosis, a disease that affects a high percentage of human beings and frequently results in heart attacks and strokes. Veterinarians are currently investigating leukemia in cats, pulmonary emphysema in horses, rheumatoid arthritis in swine, and aortic aneurysms in turkeys and are conducting experimentation vital to overcoming these diseases in human beings.

The veterinarian is responsible for research using laboratory animals, the indispensable bridge between theoretical chemistry and the use of new drugs on human beings. The laboratory animal industry is valued at nearly $500 million annually, and millions of dollars, for example, may be invested in a single stage of a research project involving germfree animals of a given genetic type. But the expense and the effort are wasted if the animals carry a latent disease or a genetic factor that can distort the investigator's findings. Veterinary and other medical researchers depend on veterinarians in laboratory animal medicine to conduct investigations using high-quality standardized animals such as those that are germ free. The development of the Sabin vaccine alone required fifteen years of research on 30,000 Indian and Philippine monkeys. Since this vaccine prevents poliomyelitis, we no longer need to close restaurants, swimming pools, and theaters during the summer in vain attempts to prevent the spread of this dread disease that killed and crippled thousands of people every year.

Veterinarians have played an important part in putting people into space by studying the reactions of animal subjects to high altitudes, acceleration, and deceleration. Their space research using monkeys and chimpanzees preceded manned space flight. In the manned space program a veterinarian heads the food and nutrition section that supplies the specialized space flight food, and another heads the radiological health team that is responsible for planning the evasion of radiation belts on space flights. A veterinarian was the first biological scientist to use lunar material in toxicological experiments.

Veterinarians are also working with marine mammals such as sea lions and dolphins to determine the effects of pressure and stress under water. Their findings will aid human aquanauts working at great depths in the sea exploring marine resources to help with the task of feeding the world's people.

Veterinary medical research is essential to determine the effects of radiation on animals, ultimately to protect human welfare. Veterinarians study the effects of both industrial nuclear energy and emergency radiation dosage to see how they affect the animal systems that we use for food. Animal tests can also establish safe dosage levels for human beings.

We depend on veterinary toxicologists to determine the toxic potential of many chemicals, discover how they accumulate or dissipate in the environment, and evaluate their potential threat to people and animals The present severe shortage of these specialists could have alarming repercussions, since over 3 million chemicals are known and new substances are being synthesized at the rate of over 7,000 a year. Veterinarians conduct research using animals to determine whether newly synthesized compounds are useful for the treatment or prevention of disease in human beings. If a drug has therapeutic value, the veterinarians pursue their investigation to determine the dosage that can be safely administered.

Fortunately the acute shortage of veterinarians in the United States has not resulted in relaxing the standards of research relating to the discovery of new drugs for the treatment of human illness. In Europe in the 1960s, women who had taken the tranquilizing drug thalidomide during pregnancy gave birth to malformed babies who were missing fingers, hands, and feet. The shortage of veterinarians had made it impossible for the drug industry to conduct vital research on animals in order to determine the efficacy and possible dangerous effects of thalidomide before the drug was released for human use. The United States Congress, recognizing the shortage of veterinarians and the resulting tragic threat to human life, passed the Health Manpower Act of 1971 to provide funds to expand colleges of veterinary medicine through loans and scholarships for veterinary medical students and funds for facilities and educational improvement.

Dr. Luther Terry, Vice President for Medical Affairs of the University of Pennsylvania and also former Surgeon General of the United States Public Health Service, has referred to veterinary medicine as being at a stage of scientific maturity, and he stated that the profession was in a position to make its greatest contribution to human health and welfare. Some of the programs now being conducted by veterinarians have enormous implications for human health. Germ-free isolators and technology developed by veterinarians are now being used for burn patients.

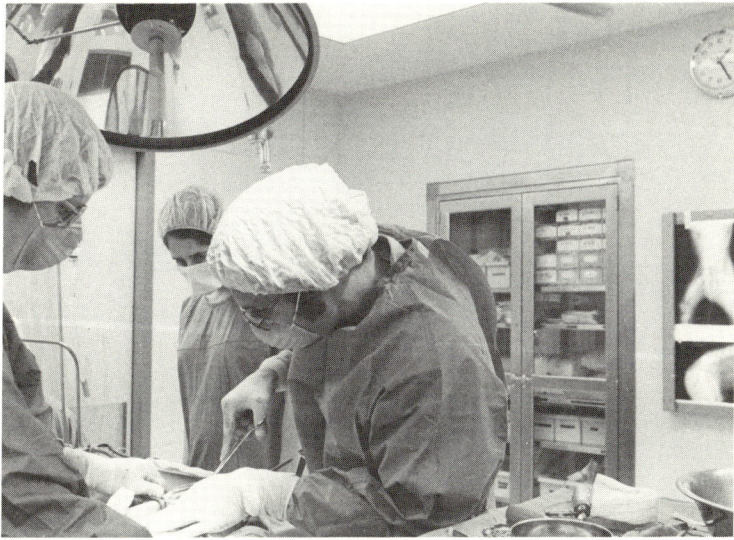

Fig. 37. Veterinary surgery involving the orthopedic surgeon, the animal patient, a surgical resident, and a veterinary student.

Some of the most promising investigative work on viruses as a possible cause of cancer is being done by veterinarians using germ-free technology. A new technique for repairing heart defects in animals may mean survival for human babies born with this defect. Research using germ-free animals has enabled veterinarians to make discoveries related to virus-induced cancer and infectious diseases in animals. The Stader splint, a metal bar with a stell pin at each end for insertion into the bone on either side of a fracture, was first demonstrated in the early 1937. It is the invention of Dr. Otto Stader, a veterinarian from Ardmore, Pennsylvania. Spinal anesthesia was first developed by veterinarians, who were also the first to perform open heart surgery and organ transplants.

In the field of animal health itself, veterinary medicine is responding to the huge growth in popularity of all types of animals kept as pets for companionship and pleasure. It has been recognized that pets make very definite psychological contributions to the mental health and wellbeing of urban dwellers. There are an estimated 125 million dogs, cats, birds, fish, and other companion animals owned by families in the United States now, and a projected estimate using a ratio of animals owned by the present population indicates that there may be more than 135 million by 1980. (See Fig. 37.)

Horse racing is a billion-dollar business, and the number of pleasure horses is on the increase in every part of the country. Zoos now have

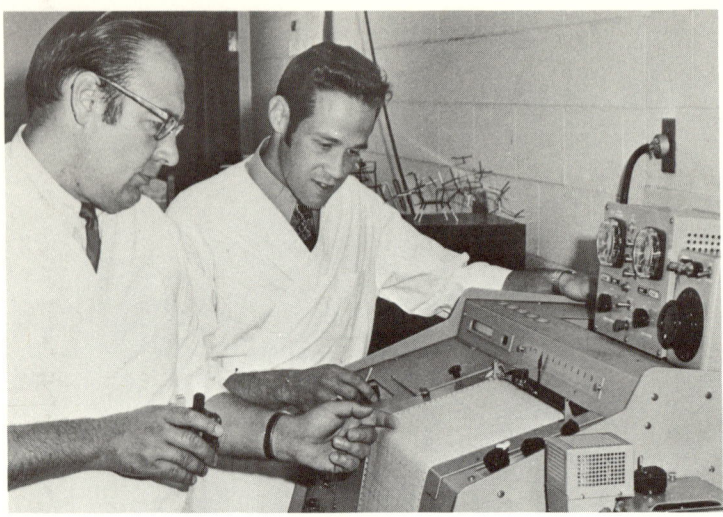

Fig. 38. The modern veterinary hospital provides health services comparable to those available in the human hospital. Two veterinarians use a spectrophotometer to check the blood chemistry of an animal with a heart impairment.

more types of exotic animals, and more scientific attention is being paid to keeping them healthy and making it possible for them to reproduce in captivity. Doctors of veterinary medicine each year provide hospital medical services for many thousands of small and large animals, in addition to making many "house calls" via ambulatory services and caring for innumerable zoo animals.

In the field of animal health care, techniques and facilities are highly advanced. Since new surgical and medical techniques are discovered in animal research, veterinarians naturally use them on animal patients before they are made available to physicians for the treatment of human beings. (See Fig. 38.)

EDUCATIONAL REQUIREMENTS

The study of veterinary medicine requires two to four years of preveterinary college study in areas such as biology, mathematics, chemistry, physics, animal science, English, and the humanities and social sciences. The first two years of most veterinary curricula involve students in-depth studies of those basic sciences that are required before they can go on to the study of clinical veterinary medicine. During the first year they study the anatomy of the dog, cat, horse, cow, and other representative species as well as the principles of physiology, microbiology, and biochemistry. The second year is spent expanding their knowledge of physiology and introducing them to pharmacology in addition to the pathology of animal disease.

The third and fourth years of the typical veterinary medical curriculum plunge students into the practice of veterinary medicine through clinical studies in such areas as medicine, surgery, radiology, receiving, outpatient practice, farm practice, clinical pathology, public health, and preventive medicine. At the present time many veterinary colleges are working toward improvements in their curriculums, and several have adopted core-elective programs.

In this new curriculum the principles of comparative medical science are taught in the first two quarters. From the third quarter to the end of the third year, the core requirements for clinical medicine is taught by interdisciplinary teams, presenting an intensive study of animal disease on an organ system basis. Time is allowed for electives, since the faculty recognizes that knowledge acquired through individual choice and effort has the greatest value and the most permanence. During the fourth year, seniors study clinical veterinary medicine. They concentrate on specific clinical subject matter in preparation for a career in one of the various areas of clinical veterinary medicine.

The curiculum reduces the time necessary for the core courses and allows more time for electives. It also provides for an interdisciplinary approach to all subjects and offers maximum opportunities for independent study to permit the most effective possible use of student time.

REQUIREMENTS FOR LICENSURE

The doctor of veterinary medicine (D.V.M.) degree is the only educational requirement for eligibility to take the national board examination for a license to practice veterinary medicine, dentistry, and surgery. Some states do not require those with sufficiently high scores on the national boards to take the state board examinations.

JOB OPPORTUNITIES

According to the Association of American Veterinary Medical Colleges, licensed veterinarians will find their services in great demand. Each graduate of the class of 1974 had a choice of an average of nine known positions.

The shortage of veterinarians is already acute and is expected to get worse. Nineteen colleges of veterinary medicine supply the veterinarians for the entire country, and unless enrollment in these schools can be substantially increased, the nation will suffer a serious shortage of veterinarians by 1980. It is predicted that by 1985 the United States will have a deficit of more than 10,000 veterinarians.

More than half of all doctors of veterinary medicine join another veterinarian or enter their own private practice. Although more than half of the 26,000 veterinarians in active practice today are private practitioners, they cannot fill the widespread need for more veterinarians.

Increasingly, the new veterinarian is offered many attractive opportunities. The basic medical sciences such as anatomy, pharmacology, pathology, physiology, and microbiology offer masters' and doctors' degrees as preparation for careers in research.

The American Veterinary Medical Association recognizes veterinary medical specialties in public health, laboratory animal medicine, pathology, surgery, radiology, toxicology, ophthalmology, theriogenology, internal medicine, cardiology, neurology, urology, and microbiology. Specialty areas require additional years of study. For example, to specialize in surgery it is necessary to complete an internship of twelve to fifteen months at a veterinary college or at a large private institution plus two years of residency training and two years of surgical practice for certification. The American Collge of Veterinary Surgeons, an arm of the American Veterinary Medical Association, is the certifying agency. There is a great deal of competition for the available internships. In 1969 there were sixty applicants for the ten positions open at the Animal Medical Center in New York.

Veterinary pathologists are certified on passing an examination given by the American College of Veterinary Pathologists. They may take the examination not sooner than five years after receiving their D.V.M. degree. Three of those years must have been spent in pathology and two of the three in work with a board-approved pathologist.

Nearly half of today's veterinarians who are not self-employed work in the pharmaceutical, biological, and food industries or in government agencies. They conduct research to discover new drugs, vaccines, and food additives and test their safety and efficacy. Veterinarians in the military are responsible for the quality and safety of all foods served to the armed forces. Veterinarians supervise the inspection of all animals and animal products imported into the United States, and their vigilance has kept this country free of epidemics of serious foreign diseases for over forty years. The importance of this activity is illustrated by the outbreak of foot-and-mouth disease in 1967 and 1968 in Great Britain that resulted in the loss of 415,800 animals. Government veterinarians at both the state and federal levels work in wildlife, ecology, space, and nuclear medicine programs. Veterinary researchers work for hospitals, universities, or drug and pharmaceutical corporations to discover new treatments and surgical techniques applicable to both people and animals. Many veterinarians hold high posts in drug and pharmaceutical corporations.

The profession offers generous financial rewards. Graduating veterinarians going into industrial or government posts may expect an annual income of $15,000 to $18,000 at the outset, with subsequent promotions and raises according to the policies of the employer.

For private practitioners the initial investment in instruments and facilities is greater, but income is much higher and is limited only by the veterinarian's professional ability and managerial talent. Practitioners usually begin their career as associates with an established veterinarian at a salary commensurate with those available in industry or government. After a period of experience and accumulation of capital, many young veterinarians will build their own animal hospitals and employ several veterinarians as associates.

Obviously, to call any of the many careers in veterinary medicine typical is an oversimplification, but since private practitioners are still in the majority, we might describe the daily routine in a small-animal practice.

On arriving at the hospital, the veterinarian might first make the rounds of patients and then perform surgery until noon. In the afternoon office hours, the veterinarian decides whether the animals brought in for treatment should be hospitalized or handled on an outpatient basis. Evening ward checks and office hours are alternated with a partner. The veterinarian is probably assisted by a receptionist who keeps patient records, a bookkeeper, a medical technician to help with laboratory work and surgical preparation, and one or more assistants on the wards of the hospital.

While veterinarians in small-animal practice perform nearly all their work in their hospitals and offices their counterparts in large-animal medicine are likely to use their laboratories and offices mainly as headquarters, maintaining radio contact while they drive from patient to patient. As with all professions, veterinary medicine demands a dedication to performing a needed service without regard for a fixed schedule. This is particularly true of the private practitioner, who must be available when emergencies arise.

Much of veterinary medical practice is devoted to preventing rather than curing disease. Pets receive immunizations in much the same manner as human babies and against as many diseases. The greater part of the large-animal practitioner's work involves diagnosis, vaccination, and consulting with animal owners as to nutrition, vaccination schedules, breeding programs, and all other aspects of herd management.

SUPPORTIVE PERSONNEL

The profession of veterinary medicine requires many types of supportive personnel. Colleges of veterinary medicine employ nurses, medical technologists, and medical illustrators as well as technicians who specialize in radiology, cardiology, electroencephalography, pulmonary function, and ophthalomology. They also hire medical librarians, medical record librarians, computer programmers, medical record administrators, and laboratory animal technologists. Private practitioners employ assistants in one or more of these technical and supportive areas. The size of the staff maintained by private practitioners will depend on the size of the veterinary hospital. All supportive personnel have two factors in common: they are greatly needed by the veterinary medical profession, and they are allied health professionals working under the direction and supervision of licensed veterinarians.

Veterinary medicine is in constant need of supportive personnel. The demands made on the veterinary medical profession, especially in the areas of research and animal care, exceed the available numbers of such personnel. Therefore opportunities for graduates in the allied health professions continue to increase. Among the various fields the greatest demand is for animal technicians.

Animal technicians

An animal techinician is defined by the American Veterinary Medical Association as "a person knowledgeable in the care and handling of animals, in the basic principles of normal and abnormal life processes, and in routine laboratory and clinical procedures. The person is primarily an assistant to veterinarians, biological research workers, and scientists."

Animal technicians are engaged in a rapidly expanding health profession that offers a rewarding career for individuals who wish to combine scientific and medical knowledge with an interest in working with animals and people.

According to the Institute of Laboratory Animal Resources, National Academy of Sciences, there were 14,000 people employed in laboratory animal care in 1970. Fifteen of the available positions in the field were vacant at the time of the survey in 1970.

This field involves a diversity of functions, including clinical laboratory procedures, radiology techniques, medical records, preparation of animal patients for surgery, and nursing care.

As employees of veterinarians, animal technicians work in all of these areas of veterinary hospitals and in veterinary research and service laboratories.

To become a qualified animal technician one must have successfully completed an approved course of study. Prospective students may select one of eight schools whose programs have been accredited by the American Veterinary Medical Association. Other schools are presently involved in the accrediting process. Two to four years of education are required before an individual can qualify for registration as an animal technologist.

REFERENCES

Rapport, S., and Wright, R., editors: Great adventures in medicine, New York, 1958, Dial Press.

Smithcors, J. F.: The American veterinary profession, its background and development, Ames, 1963, Iowa State University Press.

United States Department of Health, Education, and Welfare: Morbidity and Mortality **23:**267, 1974.

Committee on Animal Technicians: Standards for the future, Journal of the American Veterinary Medical Association **156:**396, 1970.

PROFESSIONAL ORGANIZATION WHERE FURTHER INFORMATION CAN BE OBTAINED
American Veterinary Medical Association
930 North Meacham Road
Schaumburg, Illinois 60172

Appendix A
Calendar of health careers*

The calendar on the following pages gives you a quick check on how many years of education after high school you should count on for the representative health occupations listed here. The lines and symbols show what is customary—some people take only minimum required training; many take more. The symbols used in the calendar are explained below.

- ● This kind of work requires no special training beyond what you can usually get in high school.
- ●--- After starting, you serve an apprenticeship or get similar organized on-the-job training.
- ——— Lines and symbols used with them indicate full years. To start requires special training either in college, in a hospital or special school, or in a professional school after 1-4 years of college.
- ▐▂▂ Special training is required, but you have a choice, each type of training taking a different number of years.

- □ First symbol means you can get beginner's job after college but will usually need more study as well as experience for advancement. Graduate training ordinarily goes to or beyond master's or doctor's degree.
- ———→ Your planning should look beyond minimum requirements; continuing study, after entering professional practice, is important to further advancement.
- ○ Although the line shows the minimum to qualify, more preprofessional years in college often lengthen the total training time.
- (**9 m**) Special course or on-the-job training is shown in number of months.

*From the National Health Council and the United States Employment Service: Health careers guidebook, Washington, D.C., 1968, United States Government Printing Office. Revised according to the Occupational Outlook Handbook 1974-75, Washington, D.C., 1974, United States Department of Labor, Bureau of Labor Statistics.

Appendixes   **185**

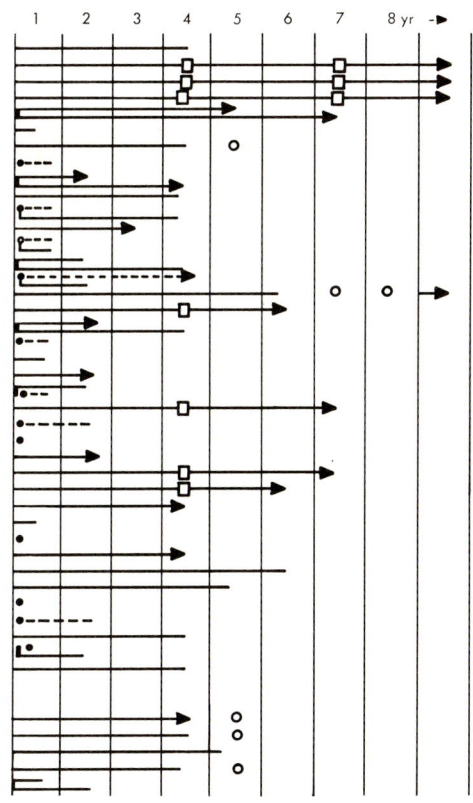

186 Appendixes

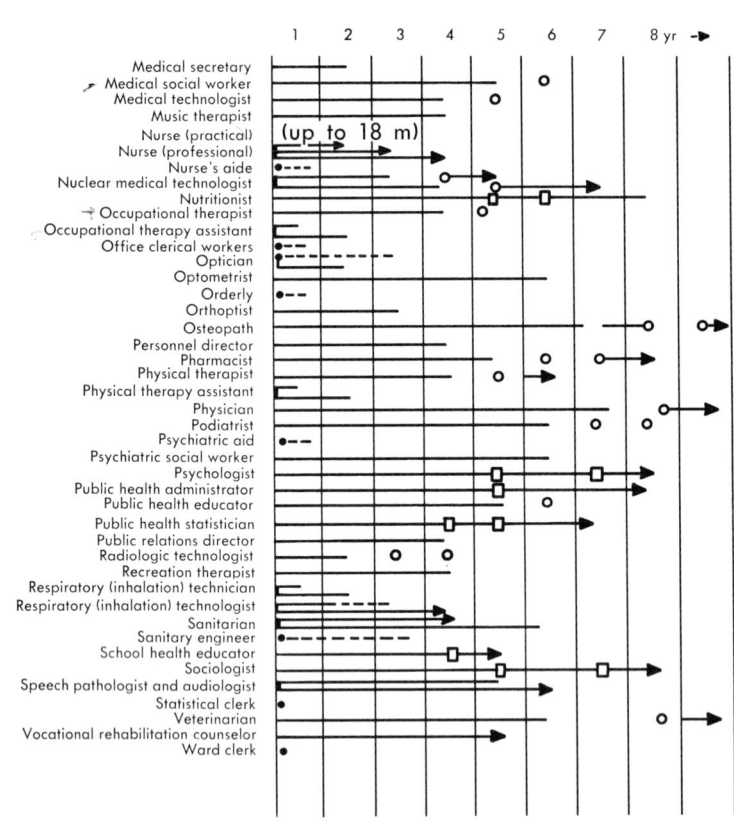

Appendix B
Related health occupations*

Students desiring more information about any of the following occupations should find the referent chapter through the index and write to the professional organization cited there.

Dentistry
  Dentist
  Dental assistant
  Dental hygienist
  Dental laboratory technician

Dietetics
  Dietetic aide
  Dietetic assistant
    (Food service supervisor)
  Dietetic technician
    (Food service manager)
    (Food service technician)
    (Food service assistant)
  Dietitian
  Nutritionist

Health services administrator
  Hospital administrator
  Health planner
  Long-term care administrator
  Nursing home administrator

Health information services
  Community health educator
  Medical communicator
  Medical illustrator
  Medical librarian
  Medical library assistant
  Medical photographer
  Medical record administrator
  Medical record technician
  Public health educator
  School health educator

Clinical laboratory services
  Chemistry technologist
  Cytotechnologist
  Hematology technologist
  Histologic technician
  Medical laboratory technician
  Medical technologist
  Microbiology technologist
  Nuclear medical technologist
  Pathologist

Medicine
  (Allopathic) Physician (M.D.)
  Osteopathic physician (D.O.)
  Medical specialties
    General and/or family practice
    Internal medicine
    Pediatrics
    Dermatology
    Surgery
    Obstetrics and gynecology
    Ophthalmology
    Otolaryngology
    Urology
    Anesthesiology
    Neurology
    Psychiatry
    Pathology
    Physical medicine and rehabilitation
    Radiology
  Physician's assistant (primary care)
  Physician's assistant (specialist)

Medical instrumentation
  Cardiopulmonary technician
  Circulation technologist (extracorporeal)
  Dialysis technician

*Adapted from American Society of Allied Health Professions Glossary of health occupation titles, Washington, D.C., 1973, United States Department of Health, Education, and Welfare, Bureau of Health Resources Development.

Electrocardiograph technician
Electromyograph technician
Electroencephalograph technician
Inhalation therapist
Respiratory technologist
Nursing
  Nurse
    Practical nurse
    Registered nurse
  Nurse aide
  Nurse anesthetist
  Nurse midwife
  Nurse practitioner
  Operating room technician
Pharmacy
  Pharmacist
  Pharmacy technician
Podiatry
  Podiatrist
  Podiatry assistant
Radiologic services
  Nuclear medicine technologist
  Radiation therapy technologist
  Radiologic technologist
  X-ray technician
Rehabilitation—activities
  Art therapist
  Dance therapist
  Manual arts therapist
  Music therapist
  Occupational therapist
  Occupational therapy assistant
  Recreational therapist
  Rehabilitation aide

Rehabilitation homemaking specialist
Rehabilitation—physical
  Corrective therapist
  Orthotist/prosthetist
  Orthotist/prosthetist assistant
  Physical therapist
  Physical therapy assistant
Social services and counseling
  Community health worker
  Homemaker/home health aide
  Medical social worker
  Mental health technician
  Psychiatric social worker
  Rehabilitation counselor
  Rehabilitation counselor aide
  School health aide
Speech and hearing services
  Audiologist
  Phoniatrist
  Speech and hearing therapist
  Speech and hearing therapy aide
  Speech pathologist
Vision care
  Ophthalmic assistant
  Ophthalmic laboratory technician
  Ophthalmologist
  Optometric assistant
  Optometrist
  Orthoptist
Veterinary medicine
  Laboratory animal specialist
  Veterinarian

Appendix C
Supply of active formally trained selected health personnel*

Occupation	1970	1980†	1990†
Certified laboratory assistants	6,700	22,260	41,160
Cytotechnologists	2,400	4,670	7,400
Dental assistants	9,200	39,110	71,530
Dental hygientists	15,100	34,190	57,650
Dental laboratory technicians	1,600	7,070	14,290
Dentists	102,220	126,170	154,910
Dietitians	15,300	18,170	22,340
Licensed practical nurses	400,000	565,890	819,790
Medical record administrators	4,200	5,140	6,430
Medical record technicians	3,800	4,900	6,460
Medical technologists	45,000	80,620	123,520
Occupational therapists	7,300	11,760	16,880
Occupational therapy assistants	600	4,360	8,820
Optometrists	18,400	21,800	28,000
Pharmacists	129,300	146,100	179,900
Physical therapists	11,550	23,030	36,570
Physicians (M.D. and D.O.)	323,200	446,800	593,800
Podiatrists	7,100	8,500	13,000
Radiologic technologists	41,000	93,560	161,280
Registered nurses	723,000	1,099,600	1,466,700
Respiratory therapists	3,850	10,510	18,810
Speech pathologists and audiologists	13,300	37,070	70,930
Veterinarians	25,900	36,400	48,100

*Modified from The supply of health manpower 1970, profiles and projections to 1990, Washington, D.C., 1974, United States Department of Health, Education, and Welfare.
†Figures in these columns are projected data

Appendix D

Professional organizations where further information may be obtained

American Academy of Physician's
Assistants
2120 L Street, N.W.
Washington, D.C. 20037

American Association for Health,
Physical Education and Recreation
1201 16th Street, N.W.
Washington, D.C. 20036

American Association for
Respiratory Therapy
7411 Hines Place
Dallas, Texas 75235

American Association of Nurse
Anesthetists
Suite 929
111 East Wacker Drive
Chicago, Illinois 60601

American College of Hospital
Administrators
840 North Lake Shore Drive
Chicago, Illinois 60611

American College of Nurse-
Midwives
1000 Vermont Avenue, N.W.
Washington, D.C. 20005

American Dental Association and
American Dental Hygienists'
Association
211 East Chicago Avenue
Chicago, Illinois 60611

American Dietetic Association
430 North Michigan Avenue
Chicago, Illinois 60611

American Medical Association
535 North Dearborn Street
Chicago, Illinois 60610

American Medical Record
Association
875 North Michigan Avenue
Suite 1850 John Hancock Center
Chicago, Illinois 60611

American Nurses' Association
10 Columbus Circle
New York, New York 10019

American Occupational Therapy
Association
6000 Executive Boulevard
Rockville, Maryland 20852

American Optometric Association
7000 Chippewa Street
St. Louis, Missouri 63119

American Osteopathic Association
212 East Ohio Street
Chicago, Illinois 60611

American Pharmaceutical Association
2215 Constitution Avenue, N.W.
Washington, D.C. 20037

American Physical Therapy
Association
1156 15th Street, N.W.
Washington, D.C. 20005

American Podiatry Association
20 Chevy Chase Circle, N.W.
Washington, D.C. 20015

American Public Health Association
1015 18th Street, N.W.
Washington, D.C. 20036

American Registry of Radiologic
Technologists
2600 Wayzata Boulevard
Minneapolis, Minnesota 55405

Appendixes **191**

American School Health Association
P.O. Box 708
Kent, Ohio 44240

American Society of Allied Health Professions
Suite 300
#1 Dupont Circle, N.W.
Washington, D.C. 20036

American Society of Clinical Pathologists
2100 West Harrison Street
Chicago, Illinois 60612

American Society of Extracorporeal Technology
6352 Oakton Street
Morton Grove, Illinois 60053

American Society for Medical Technology
Suite 200
5555 West Loop South
Bellaire, Texas 77401

American Society of Radiologic Technologists
Suite 836
500 North Michigan Avenue
Chicago, Illinois 60611

American Speech and Hearing Association
9030 Old Georgetown Road
Washington, D.C. 20014

American Veterinary Medical Association
930 North Meacham Road
Schaumberg, Illinois 60172

Association of Medical Illustrators
6650 Northwest Highway
Chicago, Illinois 60631

Association of Physician's Assistant Programs
2120 L Street, N.W.
Washington, D.C. 20037

Association of Schools of Allied Health Professions
Suite 300
#1 Dupont Circle, N.W.
Washington, D.C. 20036

Association of University Programs in Health Administration
Suite 420
#1 Dupont Circle, N.W.
Washington, D.C. 20036

Council on Social Work Education
345 East 46th Street
New York, New York 10017

Health Education Media Association
P.O. Box 5744
Bethesda, Maryland 20014

Health Sciences Communication Association
P.O. Box 79
Millbrae, California 94030

National Accrediting Agency for Clinical Laboratory Services
Suite 1512
222 South Riverside Plaza
Chicago, Illinois 60606

National Association of Social Workers, Inc.
600 Southern Building
15th and H Streets
Washington, D.C. 20005

National Commission on Certification of Physician's Assistants
3384 Peachtree Road, N.E.
Atlanta, Georgia 30326

National League for Nursing
10 Columbus Circle
New York, New York 10019

Registry of Medical Technologists of ASCP
P.O. Box 4872
Chicago, Illinois 60680

Society for Public Health Education
655 Sutter Street
San Francisco, California 94102

Index

A

Accreditation; see Credentials
Accredited record technician, 68
Acupuncture, 82
Administrators
   hospital and health services; see Hospital and health services administration
   medical record; see Medical record administration
Air, dephlogisticated, 148
American Association for Respiratory Therapy, 150, 155
American Association of Nurse Anesthetists, 98
American College of Hospital Administrators, 42
American College of Nurse-Midwives, 101, 102
American Dental Association, 9, 17
American Dental Hygienists' Association, 10, 13
American Dietetic Association, 22, 23, 25, 28, 29
American Hospital Association, 41
American Medical Association, 66, 67, 68, 134
American Medical Record Association, 60, 66, 67
American Occupational Therapy Association, 109
American Optometric Association, 115
American Osteopathic Association, 90, 140
American Physical Therapy Association, 124, 126, 127
American Podiatry Association, 138, 140
American Public Health Association, 38, 41
American Society for Medical Technology (ASMT), 71
American Society of Clinical Pathologists (ASCP), 71
American Society of Extracorporeal Technology, 34
American Society of Radiologic Technologists, 145, 147
American Speech and Hearing Association, 168, 172
American Veterinary Medical Association, 180, 182, 183
Anesthesiology, nurse; see Nurse anesthesiology
Aniseikonia, definition of, 114
Assistants
   certified laboratory, 77
   certified occupational therapy, 110
   dental, 17, 18
   dietetic, 29
   optometric, 116
   physical therapy, 127
   physician's, 82
   podiatry, 140
Association of American Medical Colleges, 4
Association of American Veterinary Colleges, 179
Association of Medical Illustrators, 56, 59
Association of Mental Health Administrators, 41
Athletic trainers, 129
Audiologists, 165

B

Beddoes, Thomas, 149
Bell, Alexander Graham, 166
Biomedical communications; see Medical communications

Index 193

Black, G. V., 15
Boher, John, 15
Bond, Thomas, 41
Boyle, Robert, 148
Breckinridge, Mary, 101
Brödel, Max, 56

C

Calendar of health careers, 184
Certification, 3
 continued, 3
Certified laboratory assistants, 77
Children's Television Network, 37
Chiropody, 137
Circulation technology; see Extracorporeal circulation technology
Colt, Samuel, 149
Communications; see Medical communications; Speech and hearing science
Community health educators, 36, 38
Community health nursing, 96
Comprehensive Health Planning, 7
Computers in health care, 62, 65, 66
Cooper, John, 4
Credentials, 2
 accreditation and, 3
 certification and, 3, 135
 establishment of, 2
 examination, equivalency and, 3
 and licensure, 3, 87, 95, 102, 123, 126
 reciprocity and, 3, 87, 123
 registration and, 3, 109
Cytotechnologists, 78

D

da Vinci, Leonardo, 49, 55
Degrees awarded, doctoral
 D.V.M., 179
 O.D., 116
 D.O., 187, 189
 M.D., 87, 187, 189
 D.P.M., 139
Dental assistants, 17, 18
Dental hygiene, 9-13
 background of, 9
 career opportunities in, 12
 curriculum for, 10-11
 educational programs in, 9-10
 functions in, 9, 12
 licensing in, 11
 personal qualifications for, 12-13
 professional organization for, 13
 salaries in, 12

Dental hygienists, 17; see also Dental hygiene
Dental laboratory technicians, 18
Dental technologists, 17
Dentatores, 14
Dentistry, 14-20
 admission requirements for, 17
 careers in, 19
 education for, 15-17
 examinations in, 17
 future trends of, 18
 history of, 14
 personal qualifications for, 20
 specialties in, 19
 supporting professionals in, 17
Dephlogisticated air, 148
Dietetic assistants, 29
Dietetic technicians, 28
Dietetics, 21-30
 development of, 21
 educational preparation for, 23-25
 job opportunities in, 26-28
 need for, 28
 practice of, 23
 qualities for, 23
 registration for, 25-26
 supporting professionals in, 28
Dietetians, medical, 21, 121; see also Dietetics

E

Education
 continuing, 3, 4, 5
 health; see Health education
 liberal arts and technical, difference between, 4
 professional, 4
Education of health professionals, 3
Edwards, Charles, 37
Ellis, Alexander J., 167
Essentials of educational programs, 4, 67, 151
Ethics, medical, 85
Extracorporeal circulation technology, 31-35
 career opportunities in, 34
 certification in, 34
 educational requirements of, 34
 professional development of, 31-33
Extracorporeal Technology, American Society of, 35

F

Fauchard, Pierre, 14, 15
Fildes, Sir Luke, 88
Fletcher, Harvey, 167

Flexner, Abraham, 1, 2
Fones, Alfred C., 9
Franklin, Benjamin, 41
Frontier Nursing Service, 101

G

Greenwood, John, 15

H

Hahnemann, Samuel, 81
Harris, Chapin B., 15
Harris, John, 15
Headstart, 163
Health
   definition of, 2
   team; see Team
Health care
   legislation for, 7
   nurse-midwifery contributions to, 102
   nurse contributions to, 91-93
   physical therapy contributions to, 129-131
   team concept in, 4, 5-7
Health careers, calendar of, 184-186
Health education, 36-40
   career opportunities in, 38
   definition of, 36
   dental, 9, 17
   Ohio State Planning Committee for, 37
   personal qualifications for, 37
   preparation for, 38
   scope of, 36
Health Maintenance Organization Act, 7
Health Manpower Acts, 7, 176
Health personnel, supply of, 189
Health occupations, 187-188
Hearing science, speech and; see Speech and hearing science
Helmholtz, Herman, 167
Hemodialysis, definition of, 31
Hill-Burton Act, 7
Histologic technicians, 78
Hippocrates, 49, 84, 133
Homeopathy, 81
Hospital and health services administration, 41-46
   educational preparation for, 43
   history of, 41
   need for, 45
   personal qualities in, 43
   related professionals in, 43
   responsibilities in, 41, 44-45

Hooke, Robert, 148
Hunter, John, 15

I

Illustration, medical; see Medical Illustration
Inhalation therapy; see Respiratory therapy

K

Kalkar, Jan Stephan, 55
Kellogg Foundation, 22
Kilbourne, F. L., 174

L

Laboratory personnel, 77
Lavoisier, Antoine, 21, 149
Legislation for health, 7
Licensure; see Credentials; specific professions
Lobenstine Clinic, 101
Logopedists, 165
Low, David, 137

M

Malpractice, 89
McGlothlin, W. J., 1, 8
MEDEX, 133
Media specialists; see Medical communications
Medicaid; see Social Security Act
Medical Association, American, 66, 67, 68, 134
Medical communications, 47-54
   definition of, 48
   development of, 49
   graduates of programs in, 52-54
   Ohio State University program in, 50
   specialized areas of, 49
   supporting professionals in, 54
   training programs in, early, 50
Medical illustration, 55-59
   career opportunities in, 58
   educational requirements for, 56
   history of, 55-56
   professional scope of, 57
Medical Illustrators, Association of, 59
Medical record administration, 60-70
   educational programs in, 66-68
   history of, 60
   job opportunities in, 69
   medical records, 61-62
   purposes of, 62-64
   personal qualities in, 68
   role of administrators in, 64-66
   supporting personnel, 68

Index **195**

Medical Record Association, American, 60, 66, 67
Medical schools, foreign, 88
Medical technology, 71-80
  contributions of, 72
  demand for, 79
  development of, 71
  educational requirements of, 76
  job opportunities in, 74
  salaries in, 79
  specialties in, 72, 77
  supporting professionals in, 77
Medicare; see Social Security Act
Medicine, 81-90
  allopathic, 81
  education for, 85
    accelerated curriculums, 86
    basic sciences, 85, 86
    premedical preparation, 87
    prerequisites for admission, 87
  foreign schools for, 88
  homeopathic, 81
  human values in, 84
  malpractice and, 89
  osteopathic, 81
  specialties in, 82, 187
  sports, 129
  types of practices in, 81
  women in, 90
Morton, W. G. T., 15
Multiplier effect, 38

N

National Association of Social Workers, 157, 164
National health insurance, 39, 89
  effectiveness of, 39
National Institutes of Health, 7, 83
National League for Nursing, 95
Nightingale, Florence, 91
Nuclear medicine, 78, 145
Nurse anesthesiology, 97, 98-101
  education in, 100
  personal qualities in, 100
  professional development of, 98
  responsibilities of, 99
Nurse Anesthetists, American Association of, 98
Nurse-midwifery, 97, 101-103
  contributions of, to health care, 102
  development of, 101
  educational programs in, 101
  licensure for, 102
Nurse-Midwives, American College of, 101, 102
Nurse practitioner, 96

Nursing, 91-98
  community health, 96
  contributions of, to health care, 91-93
  educational requirements for, 93-95
  employment status of, 97
  history of, 91
  independent practitioners in, 96
  job opportunities in, 95
  licensure for, 95
  National League for, 95
  psychiatric, 96
  types of programs in, 93-95

O

Occupational therapy, 104-111
  development of, 104
  education for, 109, 110
  functions of, 104-109
  goals of, 104
  opportunities in, 111
  registration for, 109
  supporting personnel, 110
Optometry, 112-117
  careers in, 114
  education in, 115
  future outlook for, 117
  optometric assistants and, 116
  personal qualities in, 115
  professional development of, 112
  professional functions in, 112
Osteopathic Association, American, 90, 140
Osteopathic medicine, 81

P

Paget, Sir Richard, 166
Peace Corps, 12
Pellegrino, E. D., 5, 8
Pharmaceutical Association, American, 123
Pharmacies, hospital, 120
Pharmacists, community, 118
  and prescription drugs, 119
  functions of, 120
Pharmacy, 118-123
  career opportunities in, 122
  education in, 122, 123
  history of, 118
  salaries in, 122
  women in, 122
Phoniatrists, 165
Physical therapy, 124-132
  education for, 125
    programs in, 126
  employment opportunities in, 128
  history of, 124

Physical therapy—cont'd
  licensure in, 126
  personal qualities in, 127
  professional contributions of, 129-131
  supportive personnel in, 127
Physicians; see Medicine
Physician's assistants, 82, 133-136
  categories of, 133
  credentials of, 135
  education for, 134-135
  MEDEX, 133
Podiatry, 137-140
  careers in, 138
  definition of, 137
  educational preparation for, 139
  history of, 137
  personal qualities in, 139
  supporting personnel in, 140
Priestley, Joseph, 149
Project Hope, 12
Professional organizations, addresses of, 190-191
Professionalism, 1
  impact of, on health care, 1
Professionals, health, education of, 3; see also specific professions
Professions, 1
  criteria for, 1, 2
  development of, 1
Psychiatric nursing, 96
Public health educators, 36, 38

Q

Quality care, demand of public for, 4

R

Radiologic technology, 141-147
  development of, 141
  diagnostic, 142
  educational preparation in, 145
  nuclear medicine and, 145
  therapeutic, 144
Reciprocity; see Credentials
Reconstruction aides, 124
Regional Medical Programs, 7
Registration of health professionals; see Credentials; specific professions
Respiratory therapy, 148-155
  employment opportunities in, 154
  history of, 148-151
  professional levels and education in, 153
  professional services, scope of, 151
Rush, Benjamin, 175

S

School health educators, 36, 38
Scripture, Edward, 166
Sigma Phi Alpha, 13
Simonds, Scott, 36
Smith, Theobald, 174
Social Security Act, 7
  Medicaid, 7, 66
  Medicare, 7, 66, 118
  PSRO, 7, 89
Social work, 156-164
  classifications of, 163
  in mental health settings, 161-164
    career opportunities in, 163
    educational requirements for, 163
    professional functions in, 162
  medical, 156-161
    career opportunities in, 160
    educational requirements for, 158
    functions in, 158-160
    professional development of, 156
Social Workers, National Association of, 157, 161, 163
Speech and hearing science, 165-172
  case variety in, 169, 171
  definition of, 165
  history of, 166-167
  need for, 168
  salaries in, 170
  study of, 168-169
  voice communication, adequate, and, 167
Speech pathologists, 165
Sports medicine, 129
Stader, Otto, 177
Stahl, George Ernest, 148

T

Team, health, 5
  concept in health care, 4, 5-7
  types of, 5-6
Technicians
  accredited record, 68
  animal, 182
  dental laboratory, 18
  dietetic, 28
  histologic, 78
  optometric, 117
  medical laboratory, 78
  X-ray, 141
Technologists
  cyto-, 78
  dental, 17
  extracorporeal circulation, 31
  medical, 71
  nuclear medical, 78

Index **197**

Technologists—cont'd
 nuclear medicine, 145
 radiologic, 141
Terry, Luther, 176
Therapists
 inhalation, 148
 occupational, 104
 physical, 124
 respiratory, 148
 speech and hearing, 165
Titmuss, R. M., 36, 40

U

United States Armed Services, 115
United States Army Medical Corps, 12
United States Public Health Service, 31, 69, 115

V

Vesalius, Andreas, 14, 55, 148
Veterans Administration, 69
Veterinary medicine, 175-183
 education in, 178-179

Veterinary medicine—cont'd
 history of, 24
 job opportunities in, 179
 licensure requirements in, 179
 scope of, 173-178
 supportive personnel in, 181

W

Wells, Horace, 15
Women
 in medicine, 90
 in optometry, 115
 in pharmacy, 122
 re-entry of, into professional fields, 5
World Health Organization, 2, 69, 174

X

X-ray technology; see Radiologic technology

Z

Zacharie, Isacher, 137
Zoonoses, definition of, 174

JUL 9 '79
FEB 20 '80
MAY 6 '80
FEB 5 '81

JUL 21 1981
OCT 12 '81
NOV 10 '81
APR 4 '83

APR 18 1985
SEP 24 1985
MAY 6 1987

DATE DUE

OCT 22 '97			
GAYLORD			PRINTED IN U.S.A